THE CREATION OF MODERN MASCULINITY

LARRY HAMM

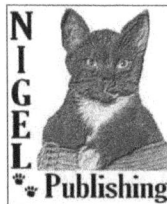

NIGEL
Publishing

Nigel Publishing

Published by Nigel Publishing, LLC
Bradenton, FL 34209

nigelpublishing@gmail.com

First Edition

ISBN-10: 0-9841984-8-2/ ISBN-13: 978-0-9841984-8-1

PREFACE

CREATING MODERN MASCULINITY

I was bullied as a child, but what does this mean? We need to understand we are bullied not only by others in our peer group but by the environment formed around us. I say I was bullied not because I was specifically targeted, although that did become the case in more than one instance, but because the intimidation I felt occurred whenever I entered those environments out of my parent's control: school, community events, and the neighborhood outside of my home. My view of the world outside of their protection was one of potential danger and full of confrontation, real and imagined. This feeling of intimidation by the world outside has never ended for me, but as each male must, I've learned to hide my fears and to present an image of security.

Females endure their own variation of hazing by the immature and threats from others, familiar and unfamiliar, and I don't wish to trivialize that experience. As equal citizens of our planet, they endure the same intimidating environment, and their traditional status as sexual objects provides them with a base of predators beyond the one that exists for children as a class. However, one of the purposes of this book is to show how for males, established in our culture as protectors and, ultimately, providers, the roles they play, like those in the bullying scenario, have implications well into adulthood and affect both sexes. The foolish age-old hierarchy that places various classes of men one above the other is auditioned in the playground. The techniques for survival learned during school days become the defense mechanisms that form the basis for those adult personalities still running our male-dominated world.

All of these attempts to become something other than that original child who wandered the first time among his peers result in a lived fiction. Masculinity is enacted as a series of behaviors based upon a fantasy of power, a belief in a potential ascension into immortality. This power serves to cover the fears that sit at the core of our being, providing males with behaviors that allow them to pretend those fears and the reality of inevitable death that accompanies them do not exist. Beneath the acts of masculinity sits a void, an unanswerable expectation of achievement and endlessness, and by donning these masks, men struggle to reach an impossible level of significance.

Historically, having males believe in this fantasy of power has been advantageous for those wishing to divide peoples, fight wars, and subjugate races or classes. Belief in the significance of one person or type of person requires the diminishment of others. For the individual, having a sense of power, however false, hides the true emptiness within that power. Within all bullies is self-doubt and fear. A façade of masculinity provides them with a means of turning those perceived weaknesses into behaviors seen as making them appear strong. This "strength" could be demonstrated in many ways, including simply being aggressive and threatening violence or by banning together with like-minded males into a gang or organized groups such as the Ku Klux Klan.

Many of these behaviors are self-defeating and potentially self-destructive though culturally they're portrayed as exhibiting powerful male characteristics. The image of the "gangsta" for example, is portrayed as hyper-masculine in modern culture, but those in this role surround themselves with others and carry weapons, two very defensive techniques developed from underlying fears. Simply carrying a gun is considered a manly behavior, when the premise of self-defense demonstrates the fear involved in this act. Like bullies, those who are the most aggressive and outwardly masculine are those who have the deepest and widest set of fears.

In an effort to explore this paradox, this work focuses on the "bad" guys, the male images that began to appear in novels of the Eighteenth Century in the form of Gothic villains but remain a dominant part of popular fiction and cinema today. The popularity of these early fictional works is tied to the appeal of these characters, and the question to be asked is "why?" Why is the bad boy image attractive and what has that to do with all masculine images? Why do females find males that transcend the law sexually interesting?

The creation of images for a gangster or a terrorist or any other negative male model is no different than the creation of positive "manly" images. A fireman, a doctor, an accountant and many other professional positions are generally considered to be positive roles, but each of these is defined according to its contribution to the culture as a whole. Each role also contains a set of attributes, characteristics commonly associated with the profession such as bravery, thoroughness, intelligence, kindness, and an almost infinite list of others. These characteristics assign a value to that profession.

In the United States, one of the first conversational hurdles encountered is the "what I do for a living" discussion. If someone says, "I am a cardiac surgeon" or "I am a clerk at the DMV," an assumption regarding that person accompanies their stated profession. Such assumptions are always incomplete and often not even close to being accurate. They simply offer a lazy way of evaluating the "other." Just as feudal titles established the role of each man in relation to each other, these assumptions are shortcuts placing a man in a rank within the other's view of the hierarchy.

What makes the negative models uniquely attractive is they exist outside of the law, so they achieve a position in the hierarchy beyond that of normal men. For the male outside of the societal acceptable roles, the characteristics are generally less defined, and, in many cases, left to the fantasies of those outside of them. As I write this, mass murders are committed frequently throughout the world, but especially in the United States. One of the first questions asked when these events occur is, "Was it a terrorist?" The label, which is generally tied to an ideological motivation, allows for others outside of the violent actions that occurred to associate a set of fears, their own fantasies, with this individual. Those affected by a "non-terrorist's" violent actions are every bit as injured or traumatized as a terrorist's victims. Yet, headlines focus on the label, as if this lack of definition gives all the meaning that is needed.

Just as the Great Chain of Being in the Middle Ages defined the role of all creations from the lowest element on earth to the highest in Heaven (God), the placement of men within and without the current hierarchy gives order to a world whose chaos can appear overwhelming. In an age where atrocities can be shown repeatedly on video, and Internet headlines of aberrant and abhorrent behavior are used to attract viewers, men search for permanence and security. Belief systems such as racism, sexism, and nationalism provide clear definitions of one's place in an otherwise confusing and frightening spectrum of others. One man believing in his own superiority because of something entirely arbitrary such as his place of birth or his ethnic background or his love of weaponry has little to no significance. However, when a culture shares these beliefs, such as with Nazism, the delusion can have devastating effects. These shared beliefs reinforce the incorrect notion that one man has standing over another based on an attribute over which that man has no control, such as the color of his skin or the county of his birth, and give the individual male an easy route to what he perceives as manhood. Believing in one's own superiority, and subconsciously perhaps one's own path to immortality, provides a great deal of satisfaction.

Gender Studies

Gender studies generally involve a discussion of the female and attempt to raise her status to that of the male by showing that women can be the equal of men in many endeavors previously shown as masculine. Though this debate remains necessary as centuries of culturally promoted and institutionalized sexism make change difficult and slow, I choose to focus on the damage done to men as the result of this gendered system. Men, as the dominant gender in these studies, have been seen as advantaged and any discussion of what is lost to them has been relegated to those outside of the majority. For the average man, however, his sex brings him nothing but an impossible standard.

Any discussion of gender, or culturally defined sexual roles, will, by its nature, include a discussion of sex, which pertains to primary (genitalia) and secondary (e.g., breasts and facial hair) sex character-istics and sexuality, which involves the desires one has for others. Beliefs that one of these three, gender, sex, or sexuality, equates to the other have long ago been researched and debunked, so the premise, for example, that man (sex) equals heterosexual male (sexuality) equals masculine (gendered posture) can be disregarded as the work of the simplest of minds. The range of gender from extremely masculine to extremely feminine, while associated with sex and sexuality, contains men and women at every point of its spectrum.

While the sex known as "man" can be measured biologically, any

5

biological component established for masculine behavior remains speculative. Though with years of cultural patterns linked to their sex, the physical characteristics of men exist in unison with their historical behaviors, these characteristics and behaviors should not be conflated. Biology creates the body, while culture steers the behavior. Spitting, for example, is a bodily activity mostly practiced by men, but this activity, usually performed as a habit, has no association with being a "man," and has every connection with being, in the psyche of the man spitting, masculine. The argument of nature versus nurture no doubt has some areas where the two overlap, and one can see where a sex born to become, on average, larger and with more muscular development than the other would use that physical superiority to generate other superiorities. To say actions are "hard wired" by biology in any one direction, however, ignores the almost limitless variety of historical male behaviors.

Gender is, therefore, a broad topic, and these pages touch only on how our culture began to experiment in print with new views of masculine behavior at a time when the old hierarchy that had simplified male roles was breaking down. Today, this struggle to reestablish an order continues, displayed in popular culture and used in political discourse. Masculinity continues to evolve, but the foundation of masculinity remains true to the core belief that one can rise above mortality by ascending a hierarchical ladder beyond others.

The Eighteenth Century and the Novel

Much of what we accept today as masculinity began to be defined in the eighteenth century when a new emphasis on the individual became embodied in the rise of democratic ideas, the beginning of professions, and the questioning of historically absolute authority. Once communication improved with the printing press, beginning in the fifteenth century, literacy increased and ideas began to circulate more readily. Information that was once owned and delivered by a select few became available to a growing number of the population. Ideas became more personal, and writers became more influential. Printing technology can be implicated in a series of revolutions, beginning with Martin Luther and the rise of Protestantism.

During what academics, particularly British historians, call the "long eighteenth century" (generally dated from about 1688, the year of the Glorious Revolution, to around 1815, the Battle of Waterloo), mass communication grew and changed as three trends emerged: content moved from primarily religious to secular, printed materials began to move from entirely fact to fiction, and the audience for the printed word expanded from dominantly male and upper class to include a growing number of women and those from classes beneath the gentry and the higher professions. All of these trends drew criticism at the time.

Fiction itself was criticized and feared as a misleading form of discourse capable of maliciously influencing innocent minds, particularly those of young women. During a time when the most frequently owned book was the *Bible* (i.e., the *Authorized* one commissioned by King James), through which the reader learned the Word of God (i.e., Logos), those romances using words that were untrue to get an emotional response were, at best, suspect, and at their worst, heresy. Even what many call the first English novel, John Bunyan's *The Pilgrim's Progress*, which came to be looked at by Protestants as a spiritual guide, was condemned by some for its fictionalization.

While many feared that female readers would not be able to distinguish fact from fiction and that they would begin to confuse the two, men were considered beyond this foolishness. Even the lowest literate man was deemed emotionally and intellectually superior to women. Hierarchically, little changed from the centuries prior to the long eighteenth century when every man could claim ownership of his wife and children. However, the ideas circulating in print would cause this arrangement to be questioned. During this so-called Age of Reason, kings heads were removed and the man who sat at the head of his table was likewise no longer secure as an unquestioned authority. Though the structure supporting male dominance was eroding, men were still expected to maintain control over others while observing a new set of protocols. New behaviors had to be learned, and, unsurprisingly, much of the fiction and non-fiction of that time dealt with how men should and should not behave. The Gothic novels discussed in this book weigh in heavily on the side of disparaged behavior. Nevertheless, readers found the villains of these novels, the bad examples, to be attractive, and though their deeds may have been reprehensible, these bad boys provided a model of behavior that could be copied.

We have now moved 200 to 250 years past the date of these novels, but we find ourselves in similar times. The modernization of labor that began in the eighteenth century has moved from the creation of factories to the creation of a digital workplace, and communication has transcended the printing press and has now become global and instantaneous. Any person's thoughts can be transcribed and transmitted worldwide in a moment. Men, who in the eighteenth century discovered they had to prove their position in their culture rather than inherit it, can no longer claim any level of superiority based upon their gender. If men could claim a right of leadership in their culture because they were physically larger and stronger, technology has taken away any such claim.

The idea of "becoming a man" is not new to our times nor our culture, but the advancement of technology into the computer age and the rise of feminism have changed the world into a place where any male wishing to attain "manhood" is confronted by a landscape of confusing possibilities. Men became the primary gender because of a genetic advantage developed around strength and size, but this advantage has had less and less importance with each technological innovation. The argument could be made that skilled communication and manual dexterity, long seen as the province of women, are much more important qualities for success in today's economic climate.

As I write this, the events of the day demonstrate the conflict caused by these changes. Threatened masculinity sits at the base of many of today's largest problems, and the extreme oppositional nature of almost every argument repeats the errors of the zero sum game that has historically defined males as men. As some males scramble to exhibit manly behavior they exhibit hyper-masculine behavior, doubling down on their historic role as the gender in power. For these men, sexual aggressiveness becomes predatory and manipulative behavior, and their fear of exposure as failures to live up to their myth of manhood drives them to not only own a gun, but to own as many guns as possible, to purchase the largest truck or the fastest car they can afford (or acquire other manly property), and, most notably, to treat with disrespect blending into anger all those who are different.

Ultimately, however, one more coerced or raped woman, one more gun, the largest truck in the neighborhood, and all the disparagement you can cast at someone of a different race does not make you more of a man. Those frustrated by this impossible quest can up the stakes, becoming violent, a natural progression for a sex long defined as hard and active (in contrast to the soft and passive female). Though originally referring to the removal of the external male sexual organs, to be emasculated has come to mean to take away one's male identity or to make weaker (e.g., proposed legislation can be emasculated). Given the demand of the masculine fantasy, founded on the premise of immortality, all men seeking to live up to this standard are doomed to fall short. Faced with emasculation, many men subsequently show their strength by overpowering those who are weaker. Beating up a smaller spouse or shooting an unarmed person reflect the attacker's underlying feeling of inconsequence yet in that attacker's fantasy, these are signs of strength and power. Likewise, men placed into a more advantageous position of wealth or status may attempt to fill the gap created by the impossible masculinity standard by acquiring more: more money, more authority, and more female conquests.

This last item seems to cast "women as objects," but that would be a miscalculation of their role in helping to create our gender system. Each of us is an object to everyone else, and while women may have historically been subservient to men, this does not mean they have not been partially complicit in the creation of this hierarchy. The notion that "good girls like bad guys" describes one way in which bad male behavior is accepted and even encouraged by females. The development in fiction of a Byronic Hero, someone who, like Lord Byron is "mad, bad, and dangerous to know," places in print the attractiveness of the independent rebel with little regard for social consequences. In a broader sense, male aggression may be seen as a strong sexual characteristic by females who shun more passive mates. Male predatory behavior may be abhorred by some women, but welcomed by others. For males, aggressiveness pays off eventually with sexual success.

Culture has been created around the human drives to preserve the self and the species. Everyone of us combines our own unique sexual impetus and defensive posture. These two powerful forces, the sex drive and the desire for self-preservation, coincide and conflict in various ways to form each individual. The chart we use to find our "selves" comes from what we see in the world into which we are born. Our current world rewards males who display historically proven characteristics, but those characteristics no longer advance us as a species. We have begun to recognize the harm perpetrated against women by our gendered system, but we need to understand that men are not solely to blame, nor are they themselves unharmed.

The Goal of this Text

Our culturally associated beliefs and behaviors "lie" on top of a lack shielded from us by layers of fantasies of fear and power. Beneath everything we are is a realization of death and the desire for permanence, what Freud called, "the problem of death." Masculinity is a way of identification to others, and like all behaviors created for others, masculinity defines a person defensively, and the fantasies become living myths. Men with wealth, with strength, with control over others have seemingly become immortal. Their perceived transcendence beyond their mortal limits (i.e., death) provides others with a hope of their own immortality.

Cultural artifacts such as novels, movies, television shows, internet memes, and political postures (to name just a few) are constructed to reflect those fantasies projected in modern masculinity. Every child ascending into our culture reaches for a roadmap and internalizes these images as he or she defines him or herself. Those young men with the weakest immediate male representation (such as those presented by absent, abusive, dismissive, or otherwise nonengaged fathers) have only those outside images of male power to guide them, but even those with the most attentive fathers are likely to be trained by their own experiences with male cultural types. All men misled into believing the masculine myth are taught to seek and act as if they've achieved the impossible.

Beginning with the first chapter, this book is comprised of my dissertation, written about something that would seem disconnected from our current world to the average reader: The Eighteenth Century British Gothic Novel. Though I work currently on a companion text, The Failure of Masculinity, the work in front of you serves as my theoretical foundation and demonstrates how cultural artifacts, such as novels, reveal a means of fulfilling male desire. The goal with this text was to establish an understanding of how this psychic mechanism works and how our culture creates and perpetuates the behaviors we have come to see as masculine, even when we view them as improper, misguided, and futile.

Beyond this understanding, we need to reexamine ourselves at this most fundamental level. Imagining the masculine fantasy gives us pleasure and makes us feel invincible; however, we need to recognize the fantasy for the fictional construction it is. Because of our natural human fears, we want to believe we're capable of transcendence, but our fictionalization of ourselves only falsely protects us. We seal ourselves with language, and only our understanding of how that language has created our dangerous world can help us to set a more healthy and happy course for our species.

Returning this narrative to the playground, I read recently of a little boy who loved cats and wanted a cat lunch box. Upon taking his purple cat lunch box to school, he was teased (i.e., bullied) into tears because of the color and theme. The bullies involved did not react as they did naturally. They learned this attitude and behavior. They learned to classify this little boy using something as simple as a lunch box. This behavior does not change when they become adults, but evolves into something more sinister like racism and sexism. Until we stop teaching our children how to be masculine or feminine based on archaic stereotypes, we are doomed to continue to clash unnecessarily with ourselves and each other.

CHAPTER I

THE MASCULINITY MYTH

This work began on the playgrounds of my childhood. While I am certain I enjoyed happy times there, my strongest early memories of other boys do not so much include their friendships as their animosities. I remember the competition and hierarchy of my first grade classroom as the teacher attempted to challenge us at our specific level, and I recall the different hierarchy that developed outside the building during recess as each of us attempted to display our special skills, our individuality. For me, masculinity was tested both inside and outside the institution, evidence my male identity would be formed not only by pleasing the Other in the form of my teacher, the school, or my parents, but by earning the respect of those others, the other children, who would assign me a value in their community. In a manner so common I now see it as clichéd, this respect would, in part, be gained by standing up to other boys, particularly those labeled bullies, whose role I imagine somehow mirrored my own. I have no memory of the actual circumstances of my first fight (the methods employed, the faces of the participants, the words that must have been exchanged), fought almost two years before first grade, but I remember clearly my surprise at the relative absence of physical pain in relation to the intensity of the emotions which surrounded the event. At the age of four or five I recognized a defining moment, and I remember fearing that my self-definition would not live up to male standards. So much was at stake.

By providing this personal reflection, I do not mean to offer my own experience as anecdotal evidence of how all male identities are formed; however, at the same time, I also do not want to rhetorically unsex myself and attempt to add an illusory disinterestedness to my arguments by creating imaginary empirical distance from my object of study. Any study of sexuality, with its need to establish definitions of man and woman based on an ideological perspective, seems arguably subjective, and a study of masculinity appears especially problematic because of the need for the male to prove himself, an act embodied by the academic argument. In other words, while I labor to expose the myths of masculinity, I employ those traditionally masculine "linguistic and representational processes by which the masculinized subject attempts to identify (with) itself,"[1] and I find myself once again trying to define my "self" on the testing ground of confrontational ideas, seeking the approval (or the acknowledgment) of others and trying my best to please the Other. Again, much is at stake.

The following pages represent my effort to uncover and examine sources of the masculine myth. For reasons discussed at length in Chapter Three, I have chosen the eighteenth century as the site of my analysis, but the impact of representations of masculinity and femininity in popular culture, which began with the improved technology, literacy, and lines of communication of that earlier century, continues to concern us today. Some degree of censorship has recently been proposed regarding the violent and sexually explicit nature of movies and television shows, musical recordings, video games, and even internet sites, all modes of popular culture. Such proposals assume that a cause and effect relationship exists between images of violence and violent behavior, but they do not address the more complex issue of why individuals pursue these images (especially when they are prohibited) or why the effect is not universally the same. My particular interest in the Gothic novel stems from its similarly outlawed status, and my examination of the male characters in these novels attempts to uncover the forces which engage and, perhaps, change the reader. In other words, I seek to provide a better understanding of what the men in these novels represent to their readers in terms of sexual attraction and masculine power, two topics which I do not see as mutually exclusive.

My examination of fictional male characters and their connection with male subjectivity places more emphasis on social and cultural determinants of sexuality than on biological factors; however, this does not mean that I discount the influence of biology on the individual. Instead, I see the complexity of hormonal makeup and the inability of science to reach agreed-upon conclusions about male and female brainwave patterns or prenatal and postnatal sexual determinants as evidence that any attempt to classify the body into a few sexed categories will always prove inadequate. The nature/nurture debate, which endocrinologist John Money has described as "obsolete" because of its demonstrated irresolution,[2] has thus far only obscured what should be the real object of our concern: the future of human relations and all of the dyadic, communal, and environmental associations that those relations involve. If our hope is to improve the relationship between the members of our species and their world, then we need to reexamine and question all of that which makes us and, by doing so, to rethink that which makes us act detrimentally toward others, ourselves, and our planet.

Recently, Thomas Laqueur has shown how the way in which medical science viewed the sexed body changed during the seventeenth and eighteenth centuries as a shift in epistemology brought about the physiological questioning and establishment of differences between males and females.[3] In Laqueur's view, this historical shift in perspective takes place as the social order mirrored on the Great

Chain of Being was being replaced by the new social dynamic that offers, among other things, "cataclysmic possibilities for social change."[4] The scientific community, in this case, stopped examining the human body as a one-sexed model based on male anatomy (with the female as a lesser version of the same model) and began to look for differences between the sexes, eventually developing a two-sexed anatomical model. Though two sexes were acknowledged in this search for difference, this rethinking of the body focused on the woman, whose "sexual nature [would] be redefined, debated, denied, or qualified"[5] because this new perspective, according to Laqueur, had political ramifications related to the need to prove woman the lesser of the two sexes. Importantly, this concern with the female body coincides with a lack of discussion of the male body, which was seen as "stable" and the "standard"[6] for the two sexes.

As inheritors of Enlightenment thought, we "continue" to "invent" the "two modern sexes"[7] in our efforts to categorize and show difference, usually by assuming male physiological constancy. My goal is to question the sufficiency of this male model and, by doing so, also to question that relationship between "biological sex and theatrical gender"[8] which is rooted in our two-sex system of analysis. My dissertation, therefore, is a first step toward exposing male insufficiency and the impossibility which exists at the center of traditional masculinity. Male subjectivity, often associated with dominance and power, needs to be reconsidered apart from the contentiousness of establishing right and wrong which so often marks studies of this nature. Instead, my intention is to show how males fail to live up to their expected roles and to demonstrate how those roles inadequately embody their sexual desires.

Because gender studies usually focus on the woman, I have found few sources which concentrate on male sexuality. As Calvin Thomas points out, "the traditional relationship between men and their bodies has never been a spoken one,"[9] and any discussion of male sexuality encounters resistance due to the anxiety created by making the male body the object of study, a position traditionally assigned to the female. "In the construction of normative masculinity, the question of the body--of its speakability, its visibility, its represent-ability--historically has been displaced onto the other, onto the feminine," and the masculine, associated with "activity, invulnerabil-ity, [and] mastery,"[10] has been largely unexamined. Moreover, the presumption that this phallic power attributed to men has a connec-tion to the male body remains predominantly unchallenged except in the work of few feminist theorists who see the breakdown of the penis = phallus equation as the necessary step toward a new mascu-linity, unfettered from the demands of sexual power.[11]

This hope for a new masculinity necessarily presupposes or concludes that "essentialist notions are flawed"[12] and relies on the changes brought about by feminism to and for the bodies of women as evidence that cultural stereotypes are constructed and can therefore be deconstructed. Feminist theory begins by refuting the notion that "[f]emale sexuality is innately more passive than male sexuality,"[13] and, in doing so, suggests that the activity associated with masculinity may also be fictive. Gender roles, differentiated from biological sex, are consequently subject to change, and perhaps the greatest evidence of this permutability of male sexual norms and gender roles exists in the almost impossible task of specifically defining "man" and subsequently finding an individual who fully embodies that definition. Nevertheless, while "[m]ale ideals seem unstable as well as variable culturally, subculturally, and person-ally,"[14] the idea of what R. W. Connell calls "hegemonic masculin-ity,"[15] or the dominant masculinity, still serves as the measure of what a male should be to identify himself as a man. "These gender ideals, or guiding images differ from culture to culture,"[16] but "in most societies" manhood is earned by impregnating women, protecting dependents, and providing for kin in a manner which tests the male under either dangerous or highly competitive conditions.[17]

In our culture, the stereotypical man who emerges from this masculinity training:

is validated by "physical strength and aggression"

is not "emotionally sensitive to others"

is not "emotionally expressive or self-revealing"

does not show "vulnerability or weakness"

expects or tolerates "anger and certain other impulsive emotional expressions, particularly toward other males"

prefers "the company of men to the company of women"

needs "other males" to be "the primary validators of . . . masculinity"

believes that women are "necessary for sex and for bearing children"

expects that relationships are not "emotionally intimate or romantic"

expects that women will "acknowledge and defer to his authority"

adheres strongly "to a sexual double standard"

categorizes some women "as morally superior, and other women [as] morally inferior to men"[18]

For Joseph Pleck, this list, which he calls "The Male Sex Role Identity paradigm," represents "the psychology of masculinity" which "our society has constructed."[19] This paradigm outlines the sex role that a male is expected to enact, but Pleck's conclusion is that this model of manhood is a myth and, like David Gilmore, who provides anthropological evidence of universal manhood trials but also looks at "the gentle Tahitians and the timid Semai,"[20] he examines the problem in the hope of a future solution. Scholars generally agree that most current masculine roles performed by men damage women and injure the men themselves, but a resistance to change in spite of these deleterious consequences creates questions regarding the invulnerability of the phallic power structure. Or, to paraphrase Gilmore: Does society demand a manly role?[21]

Male behavior has come to imply at least a level of violence, and some see maleness as the cause of the world's greatest problems, including increasing interpersonal violence, environmental destruction, and economic disparity. A seemingly frustrated Rosalind Miles asks, "What remedy for men, maleness, masculinity, manhood? First we must accept that whatever is currently being done to control this behavior of men, it is not working [her emphasis]."[22] Miles' apprehensions are shared by men's rights adherents who "believe that the traditional social role of men has become [and has been becoming] lethal."[23] Characteristically, "what emerges from . . . an examination [of male socialization processes] is a picture of considerable socialization toward violence learned in gangs, sports teams, military training, media images, at the hands (literally) of older males, and in putatively benign messages of acceptance that 'boys will be boys' when they fight."[24] In spite, however, of these increasing concerns about the unfulfilling, self-defeating, and often violent nature of male behavior, it is not changing.

Men have become caught up in patterns of identification which doom them to living this failed reality. Their models, like the Gothic villains discussed in following chapters, provide them with pieces of evidence showing how a man's desires may be realized through his control or power over his surroundings. A male character who through physical strength, intellectual prowess, or even exceptional deceit or ruthlessness achieves power over his environment, other men, or, especially, women demonstrates an omnipotence that males and females see as a key to satisfying their desires. In other words, this phallic power attracts both males and females with the possibility of unlimited pleasure and the suggestion of immortality; consequently, those characters and individuals who have access to this power and pleasure offer us examples of a god-like masculine identity that we wish to either be or have.

Morality and ethics have nothing to do with this dynamic. In the movies The Terminator and Terminator 2, Arnold Schwarzenegger played the same almost indestructible, android-robot character with one exception: in Terminator the character is evil and in 2 the character is good. Both movies and the characters they were structured around were extremely popular. Like all of Schwarzenegger's characters as well as Schwarzenegger himself, the appeal of these characters stems from the invulnerable male power that they personify. Their attraction has nothing to do with whether they are good or evil. They are powerful.[25] Predictably, Schwarzenegger's parody of this phenomenon, The Last Action Hero, in which an invincible movie character is suddenly thrust into the real world where not only bullets but also the rough action of his movie roles causes him extreme pain, failed at the box office. Fans of his movies can accept and may enjoy his comedic and sensitive characters (Twins, Kindergarten Cop, True Lies), but they did not welcome his exposure of vulnerability.

Action movies like The Terminator and its sequel provide an equation for manhood: omnipotence = possession of some quality "x" (demonstrated by the model of masculinity) = unlimited pleasure. Males seeking to embody the all-important signifier "man" enact the behaviors of these types of fictional and popular males who have demonstrated successful manliness. Characters in modern action movies like those portrayed by Schwarzenegger, Stephen Seagal, Wesley Snipes, or Jean-Claude Van Damme (to name a few) appear invincible and have access to whatever material or sexual objects they desire. A male viewer desiring his own limitless access to pleasure can, using these models, adopt one or more of the behaviors demonstrated by these characters. Unfortunately, these behaviors include de-emphasized communication skills, an emphasized physical prowess over other males, an intolerance of what is traditionally viewed as feminine behavior, and a tendency toward violence.

These movies, however, do not establish the desire to see such characters. These models are created to meet a pre-existing desire. The understood premise of the patriarchal structure and, therefore, the established view of masculinity, is that a male possesses power because he has something extra. The more of this "something" he possesses, the higher a man's position in the structure. By providing examples with this quality "x," movies respond to existing male desires. For males, pleasure in the form of received love, respect, esteem, or bodily sexual accomplishment in one of its many manifestations depends entirely upon demonstration of this quality "x." Masculine insecurity develops from the incompleteness that the lack of this quality creates. In the fantasy of an action movie, however, men are shown as complete. On an imaginary level, the action hero provides the image of a man without limitations. He is physically powerful, and he overwhelms his opponents. He does not die. He gets his sexual pleasure in whatever way he chooses. Furthermore, he is also the object of the admiration and the sexual attention of both the male and female viewers in the audience.

In Chapter Two, I discuss how, at the symbolic level, this image becomes attached to the signifier "man," and the characteristics of the image become a chain of signifiers (e.g., muscular, agile, quiet, forceful, unemotional) which are metonymically linked to this master signifier. A male then can assume the role of a man by identifying with any number of these signifiers. To borrow Mark Simpson's phrase, a male can "perform masculinity" by trying on behaviors which exhibit qualities found within this chain of signifiers. The patriarchal structure, which has traditionally relegated woman to a lesser, powerless role, presupposes that a man has something extra. In reality, he does not. However, he can pretend that he does through imitating certain characteristics connected to a symbol already shown to possess this something. Through this male identification process, masculinity becomes codified with the dissolution of the Oedipus complex, "a structur(ing) of desire around a fundamental fantasy"[26] which denies incompletion, castration, and death. Males are masculated (to coin a term) as a defense against the recognition of the emasculating consequences of mortality. Fictional males, however, can avoid the unpleasantness of having to face such consequences and can instead demonstrate a god-like omnipotence which suggests an alternative to the lack of being and castration which exist at the foundation of subjectivity.

Of course, the desire for actual omnipotence, like the related desire for immortality, remains unfulfilled and unfulfillable. Only fictional beings can be omnipotent and immortal, but these beings are included with the images which have been used as models for masculinity. Even real males used as masculine models can become fictionalized. The recently immortalized Elvis Presley[27] occupies a god-like position among a certain group of followers and has had multiple legends arise surrounding him. Some of the more zealous devotees of Elvis, for example, refuse to believe he is dead. Having given a living male the symbolic power of manhood (and not coincidentally the epithet of "The King"), they are unable to admit that he could die because such an admission would destroy the basis of their belief system. To these individuals, Elvis represents the complete man, the man who has that quality "x" which includes immortality, and to admit an inadequacy such as mortality shakes the foundation of the "manliness" Elvis symbolizes. For individuals thus involved in the Elvis myth, their own symbolic meaning disappears if this symbolization of Elvis evaporates. For most of Elvis's followers, however, his living or dying is unimportant. The imaginary Elvis they see in films or the symbolic Elvis they revere and emulate has an unclear connection or no connection at all to the real Elvis who died in his bathroom. The King endures. He continues to receive sexual interest. As the object of myth, Elvis provides a model of masculinity like the fictional heroes of action movies.

Males, in reality, can only suffer in comparison to models such as these, and, in reality, males do suffer. They forfeit their health,[28] their sexual pleasure,[29] their freedom,[30] and even their lives in an attempt to reconcile the difference between themselves and their expectations of self. Masculinity has been identified, as Freud pointed out in the <u>Three Essays on the Theory of Sexuality</u>,[31] with activity. Given the split between who they are and what they should be, males are expected to actively struggle to remove their deficiencies and to become complete men. In our historically patriarchal society, the phallus (the signifier for this quantity "x") symbolizes this completeness. As a signifier of the impossible, however, the phallus takes on unlimited, fluxional forms and meanings. Males may erroneously convince themselves that they possess the phallus in the form of a sexual partner, a material possession, or a weapon, or that they have the phallus because they are physically strong, intellectually superior, or economically empowered, but beneath this facade, males live with their guaranteed failure to possess the phallus. In terms of their sexuality, they can attain "man"-hood only through lying to themselves.

Male subjectivity, as Kaja Silverman describes it, "depends upon a kind of collective make-believe in the commensurability of penis and phallus."[32] In heterosexual relations, females, in their own search for wholeness, pretend that the male has the phallus, while males pretend to possess the phallus for the female. When the penis and phallus are equated, this pretense operates to substitute the sexual partners for their actual objects of desire. Females accept the penis as phallus and males posit the female as phallus, thereby making the penis and the woman fetish objects, or substitutes for other unnamable and unidentifiable objects of desire. Beneath this masquerade, however, both genders have a real being unsure of receiving the true desire of the other and never having actual desires met. For males, this means that each in an evaluation of his own masculinity must face the gap which exists between possessing a penis (which most do) and the impossibility of possessing or being the phallus, the signifier whose signified becomes a reservoir for unattainable desires.

In this way, measured against the standard of the phallus, every male falls short. Traditionally, however, being a man means refusing to accept failure. Masculinity requires conspicuous success in the form of physical, intellectual, financial, political, or, especially, sexual mastery. Ultimately, males strive and succeed to prove themselves men. Henry Kissinger's famous statement, "Power is the ultimate aphrodisiac,"[33] characterizes both the goal and the burden that males share. The key to unlimited sexual satisfaction is tied to the acquisition of phallic power. In truth, however, most males are not powerful. Most have neither physical, economic, nor sexual power except within the boundary of a sexual relationship or marriage. And, even that rare individual who may be believed to hold any or all of these types of power can hold them only on lease (like Elvis or Schwarzenegger). Time ultimately erases these powers, proving their illusory quality. Man cannot possess the phallus. At best, he can only stand temporarily in its shadow.

Because males see themselves as the enemy, because they are unused to sexual self-examination, because they do not see themselves as an injured party, and because they just don't want to talk about their sexual problems, efforts to discuss male sexuality have received only fractionalized male support, and attempts to change men by organizing a men's movement (to equate with the women's movement) have gathered only short-lived momentum. In addition, perhaps the competitive nature of traditional masculinity has also deterred the formation of a coherent view of male sexuality. A defining characteristic of studies in masculinity remains a lack of agreement. Noting the disparate viewpoints, Kenneth Clatterbaugh lists six major socio-political perspectives on masculinity:

1) The Conservative Perspective which ranges from a belief that males are naturally dominant to an acceptance that men will be men;

2) The Profeminist Perspective which sees traditional masculinity as a destructive means to power;

3) The Men's Rights Perspective which focuses on how traditional masculinity hurts and destroys men;

4) The Spiritual Perspective which attempts through mythological archetypes to put men in touch with their spiritual selves;

5) The Socialist Perspective which examines how traditional masculinity effects the economic structure; and,

6) The Group-Specific Perspective which often centers discussion around males of a particular race or male homosexuals.[34]

Though a significant majority of males probably align themselves with the conservative approach, most studies of masculinity take a perspective corresponding to one or more of the others on Clatterbaugh's list. These studies differentiate themselves, as Clatterbaugh indicates, by their separate agendas, and the work of writers issued from one perspective often excludes or contradicts the work of other male theorists. While my study would no doubt be categorized as Profeminist by Clatterbaugh, I believe a brief acknowledgment of other popular approaches will help to understand the disparity between approaches and the problem that male studies faces regarding adopting a unified methodology.

Current discourse on male sexuality primarily follows two patterns. Many writers, drawing upon feminist discourses, examine men in relationship to women, femininity, and mother while others often specifically avoid feminist theory in an attempt to clarify male behavior in terms of other men, masculinity, and father. The first type of commentator encourages men to care for children, support a spouse's career, share emotions with others and, in general, adopt behaviors previously considered feminine in the patriarchal division of labor. This approach often focuses on the split which occurs in men as they grow up through the patriarchal system and work to differentiate themselves from women. In contrast, the second type attempts to show male development as occurring independently from female development. This approach concentrates on what is especially male within the male experience. Both views admit that to be a man in the traditional sense involves assuming a specific role and consequently a specific type of pain due to alienation from women, other men, and themselves. While the first point of view seeks to teach men to relate to others in a manner similar to that used traditionally only by women, the second discusses bonding in a way almost exclusively male.

In examples of the first approach, writers like Victor Seidler, Andrew Tolson, and Warren Farrell[35] discuss the formation of men's groups, in particular consciousness-raising (CR) groups, where men discuss relationships, talk about the burden of being male, and release previously withheld emotions in the presence and with the encouragement of other men. The act of becoming a man in the traditional sense is viewed as a movement away from and the consequent repression of the feminine, so the act of "re-becoming" a man is seen as the breaking down of the barrier between the male identity and these (traditionally) feminine desires. Such efforts not only utilize techniques (like CR) made popular by the feminist movement, but they also are motivated by the pressures exerted by that movement to redefine sex roles. This redefinition subsequently molds the image of the "new man" around the image of the "new woman."

Using studies sometimes based on personal or related experience, these approaches do not clearly connect with each other. Some writers openly explore male sexuality in all of its forms, including bisexuality and homosexuality, while others, like Farrell, primarily discuss heterosexual masculinity. In all of these instances, however, the individual nature of sexuality limits the value of their case by case examination of various male experiences. Males also, by providing the voice of authority in a text on male sexuality, run the risk of repeating the very mistakes they are working to correct. For example, Farrell, in his most popular work, The Liberated Man, often refers to himself as "Dr." Warren Farrell, a title which he uses to add validity and strength to his anecdotal research. In effect, he is frequently and obviously using this title to give himself that extra authority that he apparently feels he lacks. In other words, Farrell himself clamors for the phallic power which may be at the root of masculinity problems like emotional insensitivity and sexual isolation and, in turn, demonstrates the inherent insufficiency of his approach. By positing himself as an authority, he implies that he has a hierarchical or paternal answer to the problems of masculinity, but, in doing so, he becomes as caught up in those problems as every other male. Though studies like Farrell's show the benefit of an improved understanding of that part of each of us which has traditionally been labeled feminine, they fail successfully to show an alternative masculinity based upon that understanding. Instead of providing specific advice, general points are put forth, such as: men have emotional barriers, men suffer from these barriers, men punish others for their suffering, men need to look at themselves and understand that suffering; nevertheless, these studies do not offer much more than encouragement toward self-knowledge to build upon. Their theme, men are socialized with a number of harmful characteristics and they need to change, is admirable, but an understanding of why and how men are socialized this way and how they can change would be more beneficial.

In contrast and sometimes in direct conflict with this approach is what Clatterbaugh terms the "mythopoetic movement"[36] of Robert Bly, John Rowan, and several others who attempt to structure a new male sexuality based upon forgotten or neglected archetypes found in the study of anthropology or mythology. Using the theories of Carl Jung, these writers respond to "the sense of lost masculinity, of being somehow disempowered by women,"[37] and aim for men "to reach down into their psyches and touch an archetypal masculine pattern from which they have been separated."[38] Bly's book, Iron John, attained best seller status and sparked the brief "wild man" movement in the United States. Using a Grimm Brothers' fairy tale, Bly metaphorically shows male growth through interaction with a primitive self, and he also bemoans the absence of a process of initiation whereby boys could become men utilizing the experience of previous generations.[39] For Bly "the average son feels, particularly in these post-immigrant times, abandoned by his father as far as soul-talk goes."[40] Due to the father's absence, males grow up lacking "male spirit"[41] and come to see the absent father as someone per-forming evil. It follows, in this interpretation, that the son himself is unworthy and destined to bear the burden of his father's sins. To avoid the grief which accompanies this burden, men must undergo a spiritual awakening by "seeking out and identifying [psychic] wounds, and by working with them in the context of myth."[42]

By examining masculine archetypes like the King, Warrior, Magician, and Lover, writers like Robert Moore and Douglas Gillette attempt to show how gender inequality has been caused not by an inherently evil masculine power, but by a masculine power out of balance with its Anima, or feminine characteristics. According to Moore and Gillette, "men of the past, in every tribe and nation, have struggled to learn how to use their power to bless the human com-munity"[43] and that the key to an improved masculinity lies in the understanding of the archetypes and their Shadows, a type of "contra-Ego"[44] related to the unconscious. In this analysis, male and female roles are distinct, just as their archetypes are distinctly different. Gender symmetry, therefore, is a matter of a male integrating the Shadow into his personality along with the "contra-sexual Anima,"[45] while, at the same time, the female similarly integrates her arche-types, Shadows, and Animus, or masculine element. The complexity of each archetype and Shadow suggests, however, that proposed gender symmetry will not be easy to achieve.

Though the mythopoetic movement claims not "to be divisive but to emphasize that there is a place for both the male and female principles in the world [Matthews's emphasis],"[46] books with titles such as <u>Iron John</u>, or Rowan's <u>The Horned God</u> have been criticized as offering an interpretation that lost masculinity may be recovered by a "return of the warrior image of masculinity."[47] Furthermore, some writers, like Ean Begg, apparently lose sight of the purposes of creating a new masculinity. In describing "the mutual attraction between the sexes," Begg notes that:

> women are attracted to men who are taller than they are; are slim, with small, tight buttocks, show themselves to be strong yet sensitive; possess a good sense of humour and a nice voice and withal are mad, bad and dangerous to know. Men fancy women who have long, shapely legs, well-formed upward tilting breasts, long blonde hair, big blue eyes, who are gentle, tender, entirely interested in them and their welfare, softly spoken and not too talkative or assertive.[48]

While Bly, Rowan, Moore, and Gillette ostensibly offer alternative masculinities, Begg seems intent on justifying the status quo. His comments do, nevertheless, point out one of the possible pitfalls of the mythopoetic movement: the danger of archetypes is that they resemble stereotypes. When Rowan uses the image of "the male [as] an electron circling the female nucleus,"[49] he, in effect, utilizes ancient types to bring about an inevitable return to patriarchal divisions and constructs a "new man" upon old turf. Yet, while the academic community has generally ignored this movement (which sometimes includes discussions of astrology, magic, and the occult) because of ideas which are, as Victor Seidler calls them, "disturbing,"[50] this remains a popular approach in Men's Studies. Although those male theorists with a background in feminism may wish otherwise, Robert Bly may be, as John Matthews calls him, "the foremost spokesman of the emerging men's movement in the USA."[51]

If, however, Bly is the number one spokes-man (or "man" having spoken) for a men's movement (which, lacking unity and direction, really is no movement), his position appears temporary because he offers few ideas which would create any lasting change. Symptom rather than solution, the mythopoetic approach merely relocates the phallus inside the male as the god within. Furthermore, though males are encouraged to touch and to share emotions, these acts are given clear heterosexual purposes. Neither homosexual desires (inversion) nor perversions are discussed. Masculinity means that men must locate their maleness in order to feel better about themselves so that they can have better relationships with women for the purpose of having better access to women. Men do not change using this logic because the focus of their masculinity, while seemingly more accessible, has not changed. Searching for phallic power within oneself is cheaper than buying a new sports car, safer than taking steroids, and less entangling (and dangerous) than having an affair with your neighbor's wife, but it remains a futile search.

For self-knowledge and self-defense, men need to understand better the identities they assume and to recognize the omnipresence of the phallic power for which they have lived and died. This work examines an historical era when the nature of masculinity was discussed and, in my view, altered. The eighteenth century marks a time when men no longer held secure patriarchal positions, but instead began to define themselves through their labor. In Chapter Three I will discuss how the symbolic beheading of patriarchal authority offers the alternatives of anarchy or this new alignment of male power based upon economic accomplishment. Driven, in part, by the anxiety created by this loss of authority, improved technology, increased literacy, and a growing marketplace combine to promote a popular discourse which both questions and supports the hegemonic discourse of the newly realigning male power structure.

Chapters Four through Seven examine key texts in the development of a new representation of masculinity. In <u>Clarissa</u>, Samuel Richardson's Lovelace, in spite of his evil or aberrant nature, displays a sexuality absent in the other, morally normative male characters. In <u>The Castle of Otranto</u>, Horace Walpole's violent and transgressive villain Manfred mirrors the insecurities of an age searching for male leadership as he struggles to maintain control of Otranto without any basis for authority. Contrastingly, in <u>The Monk</u>, Matthew Lewis's infamous monk Ambrosio challenges all authority by ignoring sexual and moral limits and exploring the possibilities of an unchained adolescent masculinity. Finally, in William Godwin's <u>Caleb Williams</u>, the power relationships between Caleb, Falkland, and Tyrrel prove mutually destructive, and each character's belief in a superior masculinity leads to his own individual form of misery. By examining <u>Caleb Williams</u> in terms of male power relations, I offer new insight into how the novel's narrative relates to Godwin's expressed philosophical purposes in its Preface, and, consequently, I clarify an ending which has, thus far, split critical opinion. Moreover, Godwin's novel provides me the opportunity to examine an eighteenth-century voice which questions the rationale behind one man's desire to surpass or control another.

While my goal beyond this dissertation is to explore potential alternative masculinities, I believe that a new examination of man as myth is needed before alternatives can be proposed. Like Godwin, I am trying to show "things as they are" in the hope that a look at the mythical power of the phallus will diminish that power. I agree with Thomas that the best method of finding new forms of masculinity is to deconstruct the given alternatives,[52] and I share with John Brenkman the belief that the solution to modern maleness exists in a "rereading of Freud's discovery of the Oedipus complex,"[53] but unlike Thomas and Brenkman, I do not offer a theoretical position which attempts to supersede the Oedipus complex. Instead, I aim to understand better the connection between the child and the man, or between the desires and behaviors of men. The gap between the experience of male sexuality and the formation of a sex role identity needs to be explored more fully. Psychoanalysis, with its recognition of infantile sexuality and ego formation, provides a key to this exploration, and literature, with its relationship between desiring reader and writer, offers materials which reflect those desires.

Notes

[1]Calvin Thomas, Male Matters: Masculinity, Anxiety, and the Male Body on the Line (Urbana: U of Illinois P, 1996) 15.

[2]John Money, Gay, Straight, and In-Between: The Sexology of Erotic Orientation (New York: Oxford UP, 1988) 50.

[3]Thomas Laqueur, Making Sex: Body and Gender from the Greeks to Freud (Cambridge: Harvard UP, 1990).

[4]Laqueur 11.

[5]Laqueur 3.

[6]Laqueur 22.

[7]Laqueur 51.

[8]Laqueur 51.

[9]Thomas 11.

[10]Thomas 12.

[11]Thomas cites Kaja Silverman, Jane Gallop, and Alice Jardine as feminists who recognize that a change in the pattern of patriarchal domination can only take place if men come to identify themselves in a way which "demean[s] the phallus." 36.

[12]David Rosen, The Changing Fictions of Masculinity (Urbana: U of Ill P, 1993) xiv.

[13]Gerda Siann, Gender, Sex and Sexuality: Contemporary Psychological Perspectives (London: Taylor & Francis, 1994) 16.

[14]Rosen xiv.

[15]R. W. Connell, Gender and Power: Society, the Person and Sexual Politics (Stanford: Stanford UP, 1987) 183.

[16]David D. Gilmore, Manhood in the Making: Cultural Concepts of Masculinity (New Haven: Yale UP, 1990) 10.

[17]Gilmore 223.

[18]Joseph H. Pleck, The Myth of Masculinity (Cambridge: MIT P, 1981) 140-141.

[19]Pleck 1.

[20]Gilmore 230.

[21]Gilmore 231.

[22]Rosalind Miles, Love, Sex, Death, and the Making of the Male (New York: Summit, 1991) 243.

[23]Kenneth Clatterbaugh, Contemporary Perspectives on Masculinity (Boulder: Westview P, 1990) 10.

[24]Harry Brod, "A Case for Men's Studies," Changing Men: New Directions in Research on Men and Masculinity, ed. Michael Kimmel (Newbury Park: Sage, 1987) 270.

[25]Mark Simpson, Male Impersonators: Men Performing Masculinity (London: Cassell, 1994) 29.

[26]Ellie Ragland-Sullivan, "The Sexual Masquerade: A Lacanian Theory of Sexual Difference," Lacan and the Subject of Language, ed. Ragland-Sullivan and Mark Bracher (New York: Routledge, 1991) 60. 49-80

[27]I am indebted to Mark Bracher for this discussion of the phallic power of Elvis Presley.

[28]Guy Corneau, Absent Fathers, Lost Sons: The Search for Masculine Identity, trans. Larry Shouldice (Boston: Shambala, 1991) 1.

[29]John Rowan, The Horned God (London: Routledge, 1987) 11.

[30]Clyde W. Franklin, The Changing Definition of Masculinity (New York: Plenum P, 1984) 30.

[31]Sigmund Freud, A Case of Hysteria, Three Essays on Sexuality and Other Works, Vol VII of The Complete Psychological Works (London: Hogarth, 1953, 1981).

[32]Kaja Silverman, Male Subjectivity at the Margins (New York: Routledge, 1992) 15.

[33]Bruce Mazlish, <u>Kissinger: The European Mind in American Policy</u> (New York: Basic Books, 1976) 134.

[34]Kenneth Clatterbaugh, <u>Contemporary Perspectives on Masculinity</u> (Boulder: Westview P, 1990) 3-19.

[35]Victor Seidler, "Men, Sex and Relationships," <u>Men, Sex and Relation-ships</u>, ed. Seidler (London: Routledge, 1992) 1-26; Andrew Tolson, <u>The Limits of Masculinity: Male Identity and the Liberated Woman</u> (New York: Harper & Row, 1977); Warren Farrell, <u>The Liberated Man</u> (New York: Bantam, 1974).

[36]Clatterbaugh 11.

[37]John Matthews, introduction, <u>Choirs of the God: Revisioning Masculinity</u>, ed. Matthews (London: Mandala, 1991) 11.

[38]Clatterbaugh 11.

[39]Robert Bly, <u>Iron John</u> (Reading, MA: Addison-Wesley, 1990).

[40]Robert Bly, "The Hawk, the Horse and the Rider," <u>Choirs of the God: Revisioning Masculinity</u>, ed. John Matthews (London: Mandala, 1991) 17.

[41]Bly, II, 14.

[42]Matthews 12.

[43]Robert Moore and Douglas Gillette, <u>The Magician Within: Accessing the Shaman in the Male Psyche</u> (New York: William Morrow, 1993) 23.

[44]Moore and Gillette 39.

[45]Moore and Gillette 247.

[46]Matthews 10.

[47]Seidler 4.

[48]Ean Begg, "Animus: the Unmentionable Archetype," <u>Choirs of the God: Revisioning Masculinity</u>, ed. John Matthews (London: Mandala, 1991) 157.

[49]John Rowan, <u>The Horned God</u> (London: Routledge, 1987) 89.

[50]Seidler 4.

[51]John Matthews, notes on contributors, <u>Choir of the God: Revisioning Masculinity</u>, ed. Matthews (London: Mandala, 1991) 215.

[52]Thomas 7.

[53]John Brenkman, <u>Straight Male Modern: A Cultural Critique of Psycho-analysis</u> (New York: Routledge, 1993) 17.

CHAPTER II

AN ASSAY ON MAN

People are neither heterosexual nor homosexual;
they are merely sexual.

Quentin Crisp[1]

Before male identities can be analyzed, we need a clearer idea of
the nature of those identities, the male bodies which don those
fictive roles, and the force which encourages those bodies to participate in this identification process. In making the male the target of
sexual analysis, however, I must necessarily begin with a neglected
examination of the psychological foundations of male sexuality and
their relationship to man as icon. Consequently, in this chapter I
endeavor to describe how men are made and to provide some insight
into the tenuous nature of modern masculinity. My efforts aim at
revealing and reveling in male insecurity because I see this insecurity
as the source of many of those lies we tell ourselves and the cause of
a restlessness which continues to motivate men to control and
conquer their environment. As our world changes, my concern
centers on the new man who must necessarily emerge from the
pressures of female competition, technological equalization of the
sexes, and the continued reduction of the importance of physical
strength. It is my hope that males will find new identities that allow
them to redefine themselves as sexual individuals whose goal is a
harmonious relationship with their world, but it is my fear that the

defensive nature of traditional masculinity will only look for new ways to establish a fictionally superior manhood.

As Mark Breitenburg has pointed out, anxiety and masculinity are often "redundant" terms,[2] and a comforting approach to masculinity which reinforces the dominant fiction of the strong, powerful male might have an appeal resembling that of the work of Robert Bly, John Rowan, and other popular writers in Men's Studies; however, this approach avoids the basis for male anxiety by joining men to a tradition of mythological beings and promoting a kind of spiritual masculine immortality. In other words, the mythopoetic movement is popular because it provides males with a way to reaffirm a traditional masculine identity which is apparently threatened by the other events of their lives. I believe that this treats the symptom rather than the illness and suspect that many males have returned from an anxiety-freeing experience at a wild-man retreat only to discover that their real-life insecurities remain. Nevertheless, while I do not wish to join Bly and the others in their defense of traditional masculine positions, I also do not wish to attack heterosexual males as the creators and perpetrators of a gender system that is seen as operating solely to their benefit. These attacks seem to minimize the female's necessary participation in the creation of gender roles and to further isolate heterosexual males as a privileged class. Instead of defending or attacking traditional masculinity, I wish to examine the nature of the male himself, without the protection of his historical made-man armor. Initially, this means viewing the male at his psychical roots prior to his full ascension into manhood and examining this masculinization process and its consequences. In the latter portion of this chapter, using Lacanian theory, I intend to show how this process which transforms a male body into a "man" becomes structurally codified within our culture.

Locating the sexuality of the male without its protective myths, however, is not an easy accomplishment. Prior to the revolutionary discourses of psychoanalysis and feminism in the twentieth century, male heterosexuality had always been considered a constant which female sexuality was to provide for and male homosexuality was to hide from. Even with the new perspectives on sexuality provided by psychoanalysis, feminism, and gay and lesbian criticism, male heterosexuality has remained for the majority of this century primarily an icon against which perversions, inversions, and neuroses could be measured. Recently, however, commentators have begun to recognize this gap in the exploration of human sexuality, and a variety of discussions about the construction of masculinity have ensued. In particular, writers concerned with bringing about social change try, through a better understanding of the masculinization process, to undo what they see as a cycle of sexual power passed on from one generation of males to the next. As Calvin Thomas states, "No social change is likely without our transforming the reproduction of a masculinity that continues to imagine its own self-preservation as domination."[3] In order to alter the sexual power structure, a task begun by psychoanalytic feminists in their efforts to demonstrate how "gender is constructed hierarchically in a way that privileges masculine subjects and disadvantages feminine subjects,"[4] masculinity theorists examine the determinants of male identity and the connections between male sexuality and power.

Primarily, studies of male sexuality exist because of feminism. The changing roles of women due to (or embodied by) the feminist movement have caused a reexamination, a reconsideration, and a necessary restructuring of male roles. As a consequence, Men's Studies has recently joined Women's Studies as an area of research.[5] Feminists have argued convincingly that men have used the posses-

sion of male genitalia as the basis of the establishment and maintenance of a structure which gives men social, political and economic
superiority over women. Subsequently, according to this argument,
men have used their authority to establish religions and political
machines, to propagate systems of thought, and to write a history
which reflects and supports this superior position. While many
masculinity theorists also attack this patriarchal structure, their
position is not as strong or dynamic because they cannot descry a
specific enemy outside themselves. Unlike feminists, male theorists
have no readily visible target of opposition, and, consequently, have
difficulty defining themselves. Even the terms "masculinity theorist"
or "male theorist" seem wordy and indeterminate in a way that
"feminist" does not; however, because the term "masculinist" has
generally developed a negative connotation by its association with
an anti-feminist position, no seemingly suitable term exists which
describes those who would examine and restructure masculinity.
Though they may share with feminists the critical interrogation of
the patriarchal view of manhood, the "male view . . . trapped in its
past,"[6] males, as the gender in power, have difficulty gaining support
for harm done to them by the system that brought them their power.

Those who study masculinity point out, however, that members of
both sexes have historically accepted, sanctioned, and defended the
patriarchal structure, and both genders have suffered under the
rules of that structure. While feminists correctly assert that women
have long been harmed by a world designed to promote male
interests, what is often left out of their discussions is the damage
done to males in this same world. Men's Studies examines this
damage and the conditions which cause it, most often by using
methods borrowed from feminist discourse. "Rather than studying
women as a means of mastery, [a new generation of male literary

academics] investigate[s] men, masculinity, and even their own will to mastery."[7] By focusing their study on men, masculinity theorists emphasize the importance of a change in traditional male behavior not just for the benefit of gender equality, but for the sake of men themselves. Before any real change in gender relations can occur, they reason, men must change, and before men will change, they must be made aware of how they are harmed by the current structure. In an effort to demonstrate the harm done to men, male theorists examine how, when a male attempts to achieve a masculine identity, to "be a man", he alienates himself from many emotions and physical pleasures while often pursuing standards of conduct which can be harmful to himself and others. Accordingly, males are treated as equal victims of the patriarchal system, and they share in the imperative to alter or escape that system. "Men's involvement in breaking out of the strait jacket of sex roles is essential because of the way it confines man at the same time as it confines woman."[8]

Predictably, scholars working in gay studies have provided many of the early examples of alternative masculinities. Like feminists, however, writers in gay studies have the advantage of being able to use traditional masculinity as a target against which various theories of sexuality may be put forth and political agendas (often) can be advanced. At their best, writers supporting the gay movement have exposed the injuries suffered by those who do not fit the heterosexual norm while at the same time calling into question the validity of that norm. By examining males whose sexuality does not conform with the traditional, heterosexual standard established within the male power system, gay studies have blurred gender distinctions and directly challenged that standard. The inevitable conclusion from such an examination is that "historical change has rendered [heterosexual masculinity] today an outmoded identity in need of

41

transformation."[9] On the other hand, at their worst, male proponents of gay rights adopt masculine power as both a means and a goal. Because homosexuality and bisexuality refer simply to the choice of a sexual object and do not, in themselves, require the abandonment of traditional masculine values, power relations are often as large an issue for gay males as they are for straight males. Jonathan Greveson worries that "much of the gay world seems to be expressing itself in ways which involve the assumption of power" and is especially concerned with the exercise of this power in a "specifically sexual manner."[10] Because, in some instances, male homosexuality represents the ultimate form of misogyny and the absolute equation of penis with phallus, what purports to be an alternative masculinity may actually only be traditional masculinity with a different choice of sexual object.

Overall, gay studies, however, have benefited masculinity studies by making male sexuality an object of controversy. The study of man as a sexual object requires a change from the traditional perspective. Historically, woman has been the sexual object and, therefore, the consequential choice as the object of sexual study. An observation of female sexuality does not require a modification of the way things have always worked within the patriarchal structure. In <u>Hidden Anxieties</u>, Leslie Hall notes that "a further argument against yet another study of women . . . is that yet again this would be the gaze directed to the female."[11] Instead, he proposes that the gaze be directed not only at the male, but at the male without the protective myth of the phallus. In other words, Hall attempts to examine male sexuality as it is lived and not as it is stereotyped. In his research, Hall studies a number of sexual dysfunctions common to men, and his findings show both the prevalence of male sexual anxiety and the barriers which males must overcome before they can discuss this anxiety. Paradoxically, the same identifications that cause suffering are often those which prohibit male discussion of that suffering. As Hall points out, being a "man" means accepting one's fate and not talking about such things. This paradox also pertains to Men's Studies. Because men are reluctant to admit to any questions regarding their own sexuality, they are unlikely to participate in discussions about male sexuality. In his Course on Man, for example, Michael Kimmel receives predominantly female enrollment.[12]

Unfortunately, an intention to explain sex roles which contradict individual sexuality often is interpreted as the establishment of differences, homosexual and heterosexual or feminine and masculine, and this interpretation places a greater importance on those differences and has supported what Thomas calls "hegemonic masculinity"[13] by assigning hierarchical importance to sex or sexual orientation. While difference exists, an emphasis on sexuality, or the experience of the body, a biological entity floating amidst a sea of social influences, would appear to offer a less dialectical approach to understanding maleness. Instead of assigning a value to the adoption of certain behaviors, a discussion of male desires in relation to experiences would better show the individual male how his desires are hindered or denied by social regulations and the desires of others. In other words, whereas an analysis of gender roles may offer to disassociate signifiers ("athletic", "intelligent", "hardworking") from a specific gender, this analysis needs to go farther and examine the reasons beneath the importance of such signifiers. Rather than privileging the signifiers of patriarchal authority, either by demanding that they belong to everyone or by condemning their power, we should question their connection to the body and attempt to determine how and why the sexual drives of males are channeled into those roles which strive for domination.

My own understanding of men, male sexuality, and masculinity begins with Robert Stoller's differentiation of sex, sexuality, and gender.[14] In my analysis, because gender studies so often focus on sex roles, I define sex as a biological distinction, gender (defined more narrowly than Stoller) as a social function, and sexuality (defined still more narrowly than Stoller) as that individually lived experience which traverses the ground between the biological and the social. This tripart structure minimizes the problems encountered by those who would struggle to separate the biological (sex) from the social (gender) by admitting that there is a path from the sexed subject to the engendered member of society; however, that path is marked with so many physiological and psychological possibilities that its study can only take place at the locus of the individual. The difficulty in understanding sexuality, as opposed to sex or gender, coincides with our inability to submit it to those biological and sociological examinations which allow for generalized observations and conclusions. Male sexuality is neither congruent with having the body of a male nor completely evident in the actions considered typically masculine; on the contrary, male sexuality often emerges in ways that are both biologically unnecessary or harmful and "violate" socially encouraged sex roles.[15]

By examining whom, how, and why a subject desires (sexuality) apart from sex and gender, I do no more than follow the theories presented by Freud in the <u>Three Essays on the Theory of Sexuality</u> and repeated throughout his work. In "The Psychogenesis of a Case of Homosexuality in a Woman,"[16] for example, Freud distinguishes between physical and psychical hermaphroditism in addition to showing the difference between an eighteen-year-old woman's choice of a feminine love-object and her masculine attitude towards that object, though these happened to coincide. Freud's analysis of the woman, which he ended prematurely, was begun because her parents, particularly her father, desired her to fit into the traditional, heterosexual feminine gender role in spite of her professed and evident homosexuality. Because homosexuality is not an illness, however, Freud doubted that psychoanalysis could modify her sexual inclinations. Her analysis could do little more than reveal the forces at work within her unconscious that contributed to her sexual nature, her sexuality. Although the woman's sexuality would result in either a confrontation with her expected gender role (heterosexual female) should she pursue her desires or a conflict with those desires should she accept that role, the function of psychoanalysis is not to restructure her gender but to explore and, if possible, reveal her desires. In his essay, Freud also suggests that "homosexual female" is a role that has only limited connections to the subject's sexuality since homosexuality, like heterosexuality, is a restriction of an innate bisexuality and occurs in a variety of ways and for a variety of reasons. Gender roles are invariably faulty attempts to categorize chaos, and they are always delimitations of individual sexuality. Though influenced by its innate biological nature and the social situation it is born into, the body of the individual finds its own unique place on the sexual spectrum.

In this way, sexuality refuses dichotomization. While each sex's reproductive apparatus limits the role which that sex can play in propagation of the species, that apparatus has no essential connection to the sexuality of the individual. "Pure masculinity or femininity is not to be found either in a psychological or a biological sense."[17] Through a history of cultural stereotyping, the labels "masculine" and "feminine" have been assigned to qualities which have ultimately and erroneously been linked to the male and female sexes. For example, domesticity has been considered a quality of femininity for so long that many individuals assign that quality directly to those who are born female. In the twentieth century, feminism has successfully demonstrated that such assumptions have no factual foundation. Masculine and feminine, used historically as a dividing line for male and female, have no actual connection to biological gender. "It has become almost common sense to argue that gender differences do not have their basis in nature but are socially and culturally constructed."[18] A "man", accordingly, is a social construct, a composite of all those masculine characteristics that have been culturally defined. He is a fiction, a model, a gauge, but, as such, he encourages males toward a certain type of behavior, even at the cost of their own sexuality.

Though the modern use of the sonogram may alter the prenatal reaction to the fetus by the mother and others and, subsequently, inscribe an unequal maleness or femaleness prior to birth, Freud's theories on infant sexuality initially related in the <u>Three Essays</u> remain fundamentally true. Psychically, at birth both sexes are sexual equals. Infants of both genders are auto-erotic, both masturbate (male masturbation centers on the penis while female masturbation centers on the clitoris), and both are polymorphously perverse, seeking and finding pleasure in a number of directions. As pleasure seeking creatures, both sexes select erotogenic zones which have an initial somatic function attached to self-preservation (like sucking). Body parts are not initially as important to the establishment of the erotogenic zones as is the quality of the stimulus, so any body part (of skin or mucous membrane) can acquire the same susceptibility to stimulation as is later possessed by the genitals. Freud uses tickling as an example of an intense and rhythmic stimulation which can evoke a particular pleasure and select an erotogenic zone. Eventually, an unpleasure in the form of a peculiar feeling of

46

tension or a sensation of itching or stimulation becomes projected on the erotogenic zone. The sexual aim of the infant, therefore, becomes the use of an external stimulus (usually analogous to sucking) to remove the sensation and, subsequently, provide satisfaction.[19]

Boys and girls do not differ in their infantile sexual objects (auto-erotic) or their sexual aims. As they age, however, 'normal' children establish the genitals as the primary erotogenic zone. According to Freud, for boys, this is always the glans penis, but for girls this begins as the clitoris only to have the erotogenic susceptibility to stimulation transferred to the vaginal orifice during late adolescence. Currently, scholars studying female sexuality dispute this transfer of erotogenic emphasis, and, by doing so, call into question the feminine role. Freud, at the same time, has been attacked by feminists for attempting to deemphasize the clitoris in favor of the vagina in an effort to show how femininity adapts to suit the penis. "Psychoanalysis now recognises that any simple criterion of feminin-ity in terms of a shift of pleasure from clitoris to vagina is a trav-esty,"[20] but, as Juliet Mitchell has pointed out, all Freud "is indicating is the path prescribed for 'normal' womanhood. Like it or not, vaginal receptivity is still regarded as indicative of this feminine normality."[21] This confrontation between Freud and feminists is mentioned here because it emphasizes two problems:

(1) We are, each of us including Freud and his feminist critics, thoroughly ingrained within the phallic system. Mitchell states that "to feminists [the clitoris] indicates an independence of men."[22] Often, what this has come to mean is that the clitoris is elevated to the status of the penis, becoming a female phallic stand-in. Though the long history of oppression and suppression of females requires a bold political message in which to begin to break this pattern, this elevation of the clitoris is at the same time an acknowledgment of the phallic power of the penis. In other

words, the danger of clitoris = penis is that this equation can take females down the same phallic road that males have traveled, both to their detriment and, as feminists have argued, to the detriment of humankind.

(2) Children have their sexuality imposed upon them by the culture into which they are introduced. Hormonal influences notwithstanding, infants begin as polymorphously perverse sexual beings, and "there is nothing either but the acquisition of this 'culture' to prevent polymorphously perverse adulthood -- it isn't a state you grow naturally out of, it is a condition you learn to reject."[23] The clitoris = penis equation is beneficial only when it deflates or uncovers the status of the penis as phallus and becomes a statement of nonvalue rather than value. True sexual equality will arrive when possession of either set of genitalia has no meaning. This type of sexual equality may be an impossibility, but the fallacy (phallusy) of a power or powerlessness attached to gender should be exposed.

Though patriarchal culture represents a rather omnipresent authority, the eventual primacy of the genital erotogenic zones should not be accepted as irrefutable or unchangeable. The existence of a wide variety of perversions, many predominant among males, demonstrates the insufficiency of the genitals to encompass the range of sexual desires. However, in order for masculinity to be changed, what Freud termed "the inverse relation holding between civilization and the free development of sexuality"[24] must be changed. The historical predominance of the penis, both in its relationship to woman and to man, must be eliminated.

The female, according to Helene Deutsch (in 1924), lives her life "under the lesser tyranny of the clitoris," remains "more 'polymorph-pervers' "(sic) than the male, and consequently has her "whole body" as "a sexual organ."[25] Deutsch leaves unsaid what she believes is understood: the male must submit to the greater tyranny of the penis while focusing his sexuality on the organ. More than 50 years after Deutsch's remarks (in 1977), Luce Irigaray makes a similar observation regarding female sexuality unencumbered by the cultural expectation that vaginal pleasure should replace clitoral pleasure. "The pleasure of the vaginal caress," Irigaray states, "Does not have to be substituted for that of the clitoral caress. They each contribute, irreplaceably, to woman's pleasure. Among other caresses...".[26] Through un-locating the source of female sexual pleasure, Irigaray is able to conclude that "woman has sex organs more or less everywhere. She finds pleasure almost anywhere."[27] By removing the sexual focus on any one organ, females receive greater pleasure from other somatic sources. As Deutsch's early remarks indicate, the cultural deemphasis of the clitoris and disregard of the female infant's vagina allow the female, as she develops into an adult, to be potentially less separated from her infantile desires than the male. The male, on the other hand, has his sexuality immediately linked to his penis, and his infantile desires related to other erotogenic zones are subsequently repressed. In adulthood, however, these desires can reappear in the form of perversions, neurotic symptoms, or sublimated actions. Nevertheless, beginning in infancy, the boy's "maleness" is located for him in his penis, and "to be a man" he must eventually close himself off from the sexual pleasure possible from the rest of his body. This simplification of sexual erotogenic focus from body to organ later parallels an adult male pattern of movement away from the potential for varied emotional and physical responses and toward a belief in simple, straight-forward behavior.

The predominance of the penis as an erotogenic zone is neither a biological fact nor a cultural necessity. It is simply the result of civilization privileging individuals who possess male genitalia and, subsequently, reacting to those privileged as males by recognizing them as empowered. If, as Karen Horney suggests, girls are immedi-ately and continuously made aware of their inferiority,[28] boys are likewise made aware of their superiority and the expectations which accompany that role. Boy babies may be handled and treated differ-ently than girl babies. The manner in which adults, especially the child's caregivers, examine, gaze at, touch, and speak to a boy instead of a girl can also vary. The mother, as the usual primary caregiver, plays a key part in how the initial gender identity is assigned. "The differences between the sexes are accentuated or blurred by maternal reactions evidenced in bodily care."[29] In her discussion of how women reproduce themselves in their role as mothers, Nancy Chodorow states, "Mothers tend to experience their daughters as more like, and more continuous with, themselves" while they "experience their sons as a male opposite."[30] Even during the preoedipal stage, therefore, both males and females are being sex-typed on the basis of the preexisting notions of masculinity and femininity, and the major contributors to this typing are the parents, especially the mother. The male infant, born into a world which reacts to and identifies him on the basis of stereotypical male characteristics, seems likely to move toward constructing a personality that incorporates several or all of those characteristics. Furthermore, as Chodorow states, boys often learn a separateness from their mother unlike girls, and as the focus of their sexual identity becomes the penis, boys distance themselves from their own and others desires. Chodorow adds:

> Girls emerge from this [preoedipal] period with a basis for "empathy" built into their primary definition of self in a way boys do not. Girls emerge with a stronger basis for experiencing another's needs and feelings as one's own (or of thinking that one is so experiencing another's needs and feelings). Furthermore, girls do not define themselves in terms of the denial of preoedipal relational modes to the same extent as do boys. Therefore,

regression to these modes tends not to feel as much a basic threat to their ego.[31]

Inversely, Chodorow is saying that men develop strong defenses against their infantile sexual desires and construct a barrier between themselves and the needs and feelings of others. "Masculine identification processes stress differentiation from others, the denial of affective relation, and categorical universalistic components of the masculine role."[32]

Only part of such a powerful psychic reaction could be caused by the culturally weighted identification which a male child receives from his mother. This identification, which maintains a narcissistic loop between the little boy and his love-object, does not require the child to acquire characteristics beyond those that will make him identifiable (and, therefore, lovable) by his mother. Seeking to return to the feeling of oneness experienced initially at the mother's breast, the infant looks outside of itself for objects to complete itself. Because these love-objects (particularly the mother) cannot always be present, the infant begins to incorporate them into his ego. "The ego is thus formed by this setting up of objects inside itself. It is also an important method of identification, so that it can be said that the ego is created by identifications."[33] The infant's primary identification, then, is narcissistic, utilizing the world as a reflective surface from which a completeness that has been otherwise lost can be attained. In other words, the infant moves from a feeling of being everything to a recognition that he must be something else. An examination of the human images he experiences provides him with evidence of this something else. As described above, this experience includes a preoccupation with the penis, "an organ with a very heavy narcissistic cathexis."[34] Still, the strong psychic reactions which Chodorow describes, differentiation from others and the denial of an affective relation, seem contradictory to the formation of an ego built upon self completion and gratification. Such characteristics can only be the result of powerful psychic defenses built on behalf of self-preservation to protect against strong impulses. It was in examining the creation of these defenses that Freud discovered what he termed the Oedipus complex.

"The Oedipus complex is the pattern of emotions and relationships that typically leads boys in our society into the roles, habits and practices of compulsory heterosexuality, into socially validated forms of masculine identity and heterosexual desire."[35] Ordinarily, boys begin life, like girls, with a strong connection with their mothers. Gradually, however, boys begin both to see their mother as a sexual object and to identify with their father as a masculine being. This identification leads the male child to an understanding that the father is his rival in the sexual battle for the mother. Then, the younger, smaller male, fearing castration from his father, renounces his sexual interest in his mother and intensifies his interest in becoming like his father. These fears are intensified by the realization that the penis, so important to his identity, is missing in the female, and he recognizes her as castrated. "In the 'ideal' case the boy learns to accept his inferior [to his father] phallic powers (thus resolving his castration complex) but on the understanding that he will later have the same patriarchal rights and a woman of his own."[36] The boy's Oedipus complex is dissolved, therefore, when he accepts the cultural value system that taboos incest, demands submission to the father and the father's mores, and promises compensation at a later date.

The dissolution of the Oedipus complex establishes the manner in which masculinity is inscribed for the individual male by acculturating his ego and bringing under control the sexual instinct. The two patterns of movement away from the feminine (mother) and toward the masculine (father) become imperative if the male is to avoid castration and assume his inevitable place in the societal structure. While, for the daughter, the reproduction of mothering, according to Chodorow, begins at birth, the reproduction of fathering, in this description, begins at the point when the son starts to learn what it means to be a man while waiting his turn as his father's subordinate. It is not a coincidence that the young male who must deny his sexual instincts and reject his love-object later shows an emotional indifference toward others. It is also important to note that what he receives in return for relinquishing his desires is the promise of power. Before that power can be attained, however, he must reach manhood, a standard of masculinity represented by the "big penis" of his father. For the rest of his life, he will demonstrate his manliness by proving himself uncastrated (unfeminine) and by attempting to close the symbolic gap between his comparatively insignificant genital organ and the larger organ attributed to his father due to his father's power.

For a male to identify himself as a man, therefore, he must not be a woman and he must acquire something which does not really exist, the basis of his father's authority and superiority. Importantly, this basis of authority must be associated by the male with masculinity and not femininity because the psychic movement, after all, is away from castration and toward having the 'ultimate penis', the phallus. The father's penis itself is only the representative of this authority, so that simply growing up and biologically maturing is not enough. Undertaking the impossible quest for that something extra that it takes to be a man, the male can direct his search toward anything: a woman (or series of women), a certain social or financial status, an academic degree, or an athletic or military achievement. In this process, the male naturally competes with other males while, at the same time, desiring their acknowledgment of his masculinity. Women can validate his masculinity only by contrast. He is not what they are. He avoids whatever he identifies as feminine.

Every male who desires to be masculine must prove himself not-feminine. This is particularly problematic in a world where the definition of femininity fails to remain static because any change which reconstitutes the feminine requires a reaction by men in structuring the masculine. Chodorow points out that the "rigid" process of "masculine gender role training" requires a male to repress "those qualities he takes to be feminine inside himself" and to reject and devalue "women and whatever he considers to be feminine in the social world."[37] When what constitutes the feminine changes, males are forced to reidentify and to become what is unfeminine. When feminism attempts to eliminate political, economic, and social differences between men and women, this male reidentification is further complicated.

In a world where women demand to be anything that men can be, men must continue to be something else. On one hand, this means maintaining male spheres of power in business, in the military, and in juridical institutions. A woman may be occasionally tolerated as an authority in these traditionally male domains, but these women are viewed as temporary incursors or anomalies. Since sharing authority means relinquishing authority (and, ultimately, the patriarchy itself), traditional masculinity does not allow for this possibility. In order to reconcile female authority, men must view whatever power a female achieves as fundamentally different or the female herself as primarily masculine. In effect, one result of the progress of feminism has been to entrench traditional masculinity within its economic, social, and political institutions. Corporate culture's "glass ceiling" is one example of how women, even as they make progress within a traditionally male structure, are often differentiated by salary or title,[38] and Susan Faludi argues that there has been a backlash against feminism and women which, while encouraging women to work to promote domestic consumption, attempts to keep them in a subordinate position and devoted to husband, house, and children.[39]

On an individual level, however, males can no longer attain a non-feminine status simply through social contract or career choice. The structures of patriarchal power (political, juridical, and social), even if they continue to subordinate women, do not openly sanction and enforce a mythical male superiority to females, and, as a result, males today face a masculinity crisis. What constitutes an ostensibly masculine identity has become uncertain. Masculinity itself is being redefined, but this redefinition brings with it both concern and promise for the future. In response to masculine insecurity, for example, males may exaggerate traditionally masculine traits to maintain sexual inequality. In an effort to distance themselves from the feminine an increasing number of males have become what Joseph Pleck terms "hypermasculine," and with hypermasculinity has come an increase in "delinquency and violence, conservative social attitudes (for example, authoritarianism and homophobia), and bodybuilding."[40] The dangers of the hypermasculine response should be self-evident, but they include increasing gang-violence, unresolved racial tension, and emphasized differences between classes of people. For humankind to progress, a new masculinity needs to be formed based on something other than the old authority. Males need to be able to identify themselves sexually in a manner that excludes phallic power. Before a new masculinity can be formulated, however, the old identifications must be understood and the myth of the phallus exposed.

Recently, Calvin Thomas (in <u>Male Matters</u>) and John Brenkman (in <u>Straight Male Modern</u>) have attempted to point the way toward new masculinities which evade or restructure the Oedipus complex. For Thomas, this means utilizing Julia Kristeva's concept of the abject which Thomas defines as "the general realm of defilement."[41] He proposes a recognition of the rectum or anus as a symbolic alternative to the penis because, in his analysis, the male represses the anus and both the freedom and lack of control that exists before the anal stage (and potty training). Traditional masculinity, according to Thomas, is associated with a repression and de-meaning of the anal function and its connection to bodily deterioration and death as the male "resort[s] to the mode by which Others become shit" in order "to maintain his masculine purity."[42] While I agree that male anxiety is connected to a fear of death and the powerlessness, or ultimate lack of power or being, which death signifies, I do not see how the modern male can be significantly differentiated from the female in this manner since women also experience the anal stage and share in the abjection process. It follows, therefore, that rather than arguing for a new approach to masculinity, Thomas suggests a new unengendered mode of representation which replaces the phallogocentric system and disrupts "the discursive boundaries of masculinity and patriarchy;"[43] however, although he admits that phallogocentric discourse is aligned with the "dominant social codes," Thomas does not show how the abandonment of this discourse can avoid the "absolute psychotic breakdown"[44] represented by another (an "other") discourse that ignores those codes. In my opinion, Thomas's focus on representational modes, though useful in demonstrating the phallic nature of language, offers scant hope of change in the way that males identify themselves as men. This type of change will come only when the body, which Thomas describes as ineffectively represented in language, is recognized apart from its symbolic representatives and identifiable images.

In contrast to Thomas, Brenkman, in his "cultural critique of the Oedipus complex,"[45] moves in a more promising direction by questioning compulsory heterosexuality and what he calls the "Oedipal moment"[46] which imposes that heterosexuality. In Brenkman's analysis, the Oedipal moment "is not at all a passage into the true biological or cultural meaning of sexuality,"[47] but a "structure of feeling" which takes its shape from modern patriarchy.[48] By pointing out how the " 'simple positive Oedipus complex' is itself elusive, rare, even a theoretical fiction,"[49] Brenkman suggests that new male sexualities exist beyond accepted societal norms, but he does not suggest what those sexualities might be. Still, his discussion of the connection between the Oedipal conflict, society, and modern masculinity perceptively targets the foundations of male identity, and his effort to expose the fictive link between that identity and the male body is an important first step toward change.

Like Thomas and Brenkman, I do not propose to know what new masculinities could be constructed from the ashes of a deconstructed phallic male, but I examine the structure of existing modern masculinity in an attempt to find a direction away from what I see as an oppressive system which requires male domination. I share with Thomas the view that male domination is an effort to assuage male anxiety with the myth of the phallus and with Brenkman the idea that change can be affected through a recognition of that myth. The problem is to understand how individual sexuality creates and is created by culture, or, in other words, how the Oedipus complex becomes the instrument by which men are made. The work of Jacques Lacan, by returning to Freud's theories from a structural standpoint, allows for a better understanding of the link between sexuality and culture, and an examination of cultural artifacts (like literature) from a Lacanian perspective offers potential insights into the structuring and re-structuring of masculinity.

"Lacan," in the words of Jacqueline Rose, "argued that psychoanalysis should not try to produce 'male' and 'female' as complementary entities, sure of each other and of their own identity, but should expose the fantasy on which this notion rests."[50] Before males and females encounter the polarizing constructions of civilization no difference exists in the sexuality of the individual. "In the psyche, there is nothing by which the subject may situate himself as a male or female being."[51] Upon entrance into culture, primarily through the adoption of language, the individual encounters the limits of sexuality imposed by that culture. Lacan understands this passage into a world of symbolic meaning structured by others as the source of conflict between infantile sexuality and gender identity that Freud had observed. "The ways of what one must do as man or as woman are entirely abandoned to the drama, to the scenario, which is placed in the field of the Other -- which, strictly speaking, is the Oedipus complex."[52] "The human being has always to learn from scratch from the Other what he has to do, as man or as woman."[53] For Lacan, the Oedipal drama is not necessarily acted out between a child and her/his parents, but instead makes its impact in the relationship between the subject and her/his psychic surroundings. The sexual identity known as "man" and portrayed in the guise of masculinity, therefore, is not inherent in a male child but is assumed by the child as the price of socialization. In the realm of the Other, then, the child must come to terms with the phallus. The phallus, as Lacan describes it, is "not a phantasy," nor "an object," nor "even less the organ"[54] but "a signifier"[55] that appears at the locus of the lack, "the advent of desire."[56] Lacan describes the phallus as involved in both the identification process and desire, and thereby emphasizes the complexity of the subject's relationship with the Other. This is not simply the donning of an identity given to us by our surroundings; psychically, there is much more at work here.

Identification begins with what Lacan calls the mirror stage when the subject (child) begins to forge an ego based upon images outside of himself or herself. The subject "identifies himself with the visual Gestalt of his own body"[57] which contrasts with an actual "still very profound lack of co-ordination.[58]" By constructing an imaginary unity (an ideal ego) of himself or herself from another (an other), the subject presupposes his/her own completion in the world of the other and "fixes upon himself an image that alienates him from himself."[59] In other words, the initial identity of the child is spatial and visual, and the need for this identity arises from the child's own recognized incompleteness, his "fragmented body"[60] which will always be something less than the image s/he constructs for her/himself. However, this imaginary identity, constructed from local visual images (mother, father, siblings, etc.), is later complicated to an even greater extent by the subject's acquisition of language and the cultural influences associated with language.[61]

Initially, the subject's relationship with the other is one of Demand (represented as S<>D) which is only partially satisfied because this demand includes a longing for "recognition that will in some way make up for the child's fundamental want-of-being."[62] Subjects, therefore, seek an Other who can identify them for themselves and whom they can privilege with the potential for withholding and providing satisfaction. Subjects find this Other in the Other's language, which promises to provide subjects with what they feel themselves denied or separated from. It is in the place of the Other, then, that the subject locates her or his desire, and it is through language that she or he realizes (recognizes/creates) this desire.

Desire is that which is manifested in the interval that demand hollows within itself, in as much as the subject, in articulating the signifying chain, brings to light the want-to-be, together with the appeal to receive the complement from the Other, if the Other, the locus of speech, is also the locus of this want, or lack.[63]

Individual subjects, unsatisfied in their demands, reach outward and grab at a signifier, a signifier which seemingly holds what the subject does not have, a signifier which will identify the subject by what she or he represents, a signifier, known as the phallus, which signifies and masks for the subject the empty impossibility of desire. This process can be charted as follows:

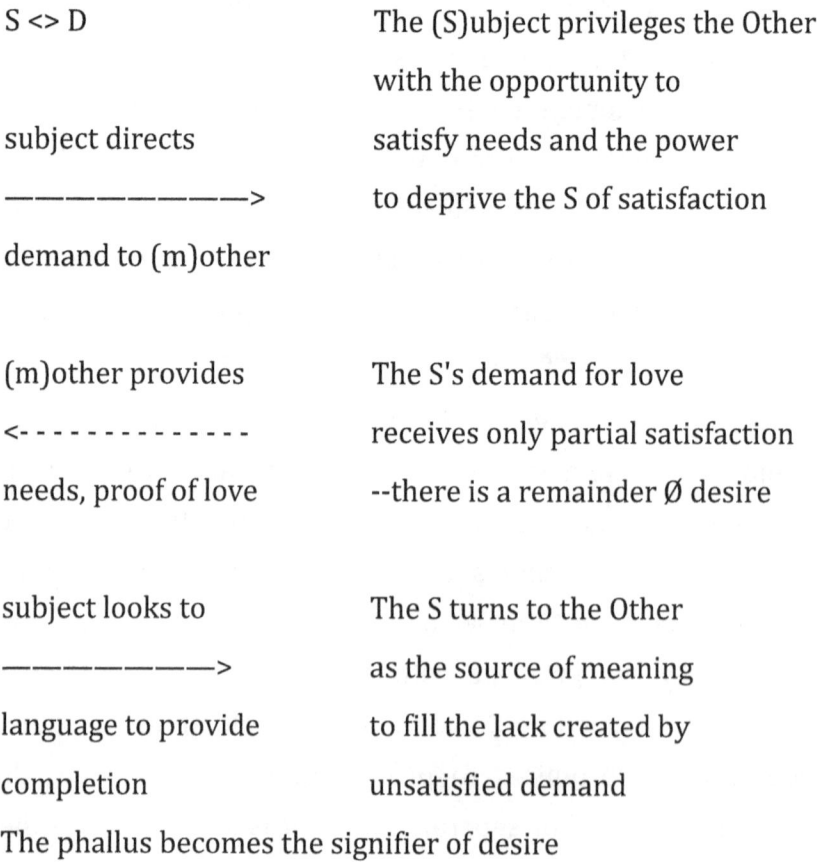

S <> D	The (S)ubject privileges the Other
	with the opportunity to
subject directs	satisfy needs and the power
—————————>	to deprive the S of satisfaction
demand to (m)other	
(m)other provides	The S's demand for love
<- - - - - - - - - - - - - -	receives only partial satisfaction
needs, proof of love	--there is a remainder Ø desire
subject looks to	The S turns to the Other
—————————>	as the source of meaning
language to provide	to fill the lack created by
completion	unsatisfied demand

The phallus becomes the signifier of desire

Desire, therefore, originates with its signification. "Man's desire is the desire of the Other"[64] or desire for and by the Other because subjects believe they can have completion if they find within the Other what they lack and they can be completed if they are that which the Other desires. With the subject's acquisition of and by language, the subject is now able to try fruitlessly to give meaning to the lack she or he feels and to search in the Other for that something she or he has lost. It is in this field of the Other where the Oedipal identification takes place.

The significance of the Oedipus complex, for Lacan, is structural. To be able to identify himself within the Symbolic Order of language the child must assume the Name-of-the-Father. The father in the Oedipal situation is not, in this analysis, the biological father, but a symbolic father whose importance includes the function of Law in the form of kinship relations. In addition, the Name-of-the-Father structures the symbols which represent, for example, one's own body, birth, life, and death. Using signifiers, the subject constructs a symbolic self, an ego ideal, and "the ultimate point de capiton, the signifier that fixes the meaning of the signifying chains of every subject's discourse,"[65] which is the phallus. The phallus is not the penis, but the patriarchal nature of cultural taboos and restrictions associates this signifier with the male power structure, making even the language which transmits culture male in nature.

The subject's relationship to this ultimate signifier determines her or his sexuality. Both sexes can line up on either side of the phallus, structurally forming male and female homosexuality and heterosexuality. "Sexual difference is then assigned according to whether individual subjects do or do not possess the phallus."[66] A male must either accept having the phallus for normative heterosexuality or choose to be the phallus (the negative Oedipus complex) which places him on the side of homosexuality. In the case of heterosexuality, he decides to avoid the castration which he intuits that his mother has experienced and to identify with the father as the one having the phallus. The alternative position of homosexuality is an identification with the mother as the phallus for the father. "The castration complex is the instance of the humanisation of the child in its sexual difference."[67] Whichever sexuality the male subject embraces, he denies himself the pleasures which exist outside of that position.

Immersion into the Other's language, therefore, moves the male subject from a narcissistic certainty into a state whose very existence as symbolic representation (and not being) evidences uncertainty. He will henceforth experience a fundamental split between the imaginary *moi* (ego) he has constructed through the *meconnaissance* (misrecognition) of outside images and the symbolic *je* (I) which discloses the subject's incompleteness while at the same time attempting to locate the missing object in the world of the Other. The alienated subject now hopelessly searches for this lost object in the Imaginary (images), the Symbolic (signifiers), and in that which is not available in the imagined or symbolized, the level which Lacan calls the Real. The Real, in effect, is that which existed before symbolization that comes into being through symbolization. In other words, a signifier makes present the gap which is the Real, and the law of signifiers, the Symbolic Order, structures the Real as the hole which defies signification. Lacan identifies the missing object in the Real as the object a, the object which is left out of the Symbolic Order but which promises to provide completeness of being or *jouissance* (enjoyment in a transgressive sexual sense).

All desire is desire of the Other because the alienated (or split) subject hopes to locate the object a in the Other or to have the Other provide evidence that the object a is within the subject himself. "Thus in addition to being the object around which the partial drives and their *jouissances* turn, the object a, as the representative of our lost immortality and vitality in general, is the cause of all desire, desire being precisely a function of our lack of being."[68] Lacan defines the split subject's relationship to the object a as fantasy ($ <> a). "Fantasy appears, then, as an answer to *'Che vuoi?'*, to the unbearable enigma of the desire of the Other, of the lack in the Other; but it is at the same time fantasy itself which, so to speak, provides the co-ordinates of our desire -- which constructs the frame enabling us to desire some-thing."[69] Fantasy, in other words, hides our mortality or lack of being from us, but beneath this quest for the unobtainable object of desire, we continue to experience that lack which we expect the missing object to satisfy, and we are directed in our search by an Other whom we privilege with the power to identify what will complete us.

Desire, the search for the object a, occurs in what Lacan calls "the three registers of subjectivity": the Imaginary, the Symbolic, and the Real.[70] Consequently, to "be a man" not only requires a male to assume the culturally identifiable body image of a man as well as embodying the appropriate signifiers (virile, courageous, independ-ent, potentially violent, etc.), but also to adopt manly fantasies. Because, however, the nature of fantasy is to pursue that which is left out, what constitutes the object a is illusory. For example, in the primary phallic equation, "The Woman" operates as the object a of heterosexual male desire, but each woman fails to provide the enjoyment that The Woman promises. The *jouissance* received from the body of a woman is only partially enjoyed and may, in itself, be unsatisfying (though still experienced as *jouissance*) because this *jouissance* excludes the *plus-de-jouir*, a surplus-of-enjoying which always remains left out. Fantasy, like imaginary solidarity or symbolic wholeness, proves ultimately unfulfilling. In this way, all subjectivity involves an inevitably futile effort to attain completeness, but male subjectivity, with its culturally-linked emphasis on activity and competitive triumph, associates this failure with the annihilation of identity. If being a man means possessing the phallus (or being complete), then each male must convince himself that he is fictionally whole, or he must enact an identity other than manhood.

Male identity gets acted out, accordingly, in an attempt to solve the riddle of desire and establish the male subject as the one in possession of the phallus. In the words of Kaja Silverman, "identity and desire are so complexly imbricated that neither can be explained without recourse to the other."[71] Male subjectivity, linked to possession of the phallus, the signifier for the unsignifiable object a, manifests itself in a variety of vain attempts to locate and possess the missing object; however, because this object is by definition something which has been cut-off or prohibited, the search for complete maleness often takes place beyond established cultural boundaries. Since the object a is found outside of the normal resources of the Imaginary and Symbolic, to possess the phallus means to be superior to social limits or above the Law. Subsequently, while what Silverman calls the "dominant fiction," or lived ideology,[72] is a structure based on a phallus/penis equation and the Law is a phallic construction using images and signifiers rooted in the signifier "phallus", male subjectivity often leads the male to exceed that Law and to locate a *jouissance* or an object a somewhere else. Though how to be a man is something the male learns from his cultural surroundings, it is important to note that his masculine identity does not come about only by obeying cultural laws. Indeed, the impossibility of fulfilling the demands of phallic masculinity creates a need to go beyond the known and the legal. On one hand, this need to transcend limits encourages inventiveness and a questioning of unjust authority; on the other hand, it is embodied by imperialism and criminal activity.

The problem of male anxiety, as Thomas points out, is tied to a patriarchal structure which has always de-meaned (taken meaning away from) women and sought to maintain male domination;73 furthermore, as males attempt to exceed who they are to become that something else which will bring them closer to phallic complete- ness, male anxiety can be linked to colonization, empiricism, and political revolution. I see it as no coincidence that these historical movements intensified at approximately the same time period of Western civilization. This is not only a result, however, of an adapta- tion of identities to a slowly changing dominant fiction of masculinity but evidence of a stronger force of male desire seeking to satisfy itself by altering its world. Accordingly, our efforts to understand masculinity must go beyond an analysis of gender formations, those primary male identities promoted, in one example, by the develop- ment of professions and supported by a proliferation of institutions, and attempt to uncover the psychical forces which directed males to become the inventors, colonizers, and conquistadors who played a significant part in shaping our current world.

In the pages which follow, my emphasis on the eighteenth century coincides with what I believe is a revolution in male subjectivity which takes place at that time. In my view (and I now borrow some of Thomas's language to express my idea), the explosion of discourse which accompanies this historically dramatic reassessment of manhood arises from a male anxiety which must redefine 'man' (to "masculate" him) in order to retain the image of phallic authority which had been damaged by attacks on the patriarchal throne. The resultant male representations of capitalist and entrepreneur, explorer and exploiter, as well as professional soldier, lawyer, or doctor (to name a few) all offer potential phallic power, but all, of course, ultimately fail to provide the individual with completeness. At the same time that male gender roles were arguably intensifying the subordination of the female, they were continuing a process of masculinization that restricts and directs male sexuality while allowing for a growing variety of economic and social functions. Men were provided an ostensible freedom of opportunity which was denied to women, but this freedom coincided with an increased emphasis on male accomplishment and the corresponding consequences of male failure as well as a broadening of prohibitions against male homosexuality. The primary proof that this mirage of power had substance was the female, whose condition was always secondary to the male's and whose maintained inferiority secured male dominance.

I will also examine why male insecurity increases during the eighteenth century and why a proliferation of discourse about sex and gender roles takes place at that time. I will also try to show why a traditional male identity (or the dominant fiction of masculinity) which has been discussed in this chapter becomes increasingly important at a time when hereditary divisions between individuals were being epistemologically dismantled. During the eighteenth century, when writers like Samuel Richardson sought to portray a new type of man who would display a virtue which would earn him his position as head of the household, the wish to identify a superior male created more than an examination of the virtuous. Males like the libertine Lovelace in Richardson's <u>Clarissa</u> and the later Gothic villains of Walpole, Lewis, and Godwin all offered readers sexually interesting male alternatives to consider. While few would laud or agree with the behavior of these villainous males, many could see their ingenuity, perseverance, individuality, and single-mindedness as attractive characteristics and their ability to get what they want as a desirable quality. Because the audience reacts not only to the physical image and the symbolic status of these men but also to this presence of male desire, these models of masculinity offer themselves as potential solutions to that lack of manhood which every male experiences at some level. By examining these male types, perhaps we can learn something about the seductive qualities of the solitary man outside of the law who takes what he desires because he appears innately superior to other men; furthermore, perhaps we can begin a course which will expose the illusion of phallic power, and, in turn, locate a new masculinity somewhere else.

Notes

[1] Quentin Crisp, introduction, Quentin Crisp's Book of Quotations: 1000 Observations on Life and Love by, for, and About Gay Men and Women, ed. Amy Appleby (New York: Macmillan, 1989) vii.

[2] Mark Breitenburg, Anxious Masculinity in Early Modern England (Cambridge: Cambridge UP, 1996) 1.

[3] Calvin Thomas, Male Matters: Masculinity, Anxiety, and the Male Body on the Line (Urbana: U of Ill P, 1996) 17.

[4] Patricia Elliot, From Mastery to Analysis: Theories of Gender in Psychoanalytic Feminism (Ithaca: Cornell UP, 1991) 231-232.

[5] Michael Kimmel, "Changing Men," Changing Men: New Directions in Research on Men and Masculinity, ed. Kimmel (Newbury Park: Sage, 1987) 1-24.

[6] David Rosen, preface, The Changing Fictions of Masculinity (Urbana: U of Ill P, 1993) xii.

[7] Jane Gallop, Around 1981: Academic Feminist Literary Theory (New York: Routledge, 1992) 242.

[8] Warren Farrell, The Liberated Man (New York: Bantam, 1974) 8.

[9] Gregory M. Herek, "Reformulating the Male Role," Changing Men: New Directions in Research on Men and Masculinity, ed. Michael Kimmel (Newbury Park: Sage, 1987) 73.

[10]Jonathan Greveson, "Health or Home," Men, Sex and Relationships, ed. Victor J. Seidler (London: Routledge, 1992) 111.

[11]Leslie Hall, Hidden Anxieties (Cambridge: Polity P, 1991) 11.

[12]Michael Kimmel, "Teaching a Course on Man," Changing Men: New Directions in Research on Men and Masculinity, ed. Kimmel (Newbury Park: Sage, 1987) 283.

[13]Thomas 17.

[14]Robert J. Stoller, Sex and Gender: The Development of Masculinity and Feminity, vol. 1 (New York: Jason Aronson, 1968, 1974).

[15]Rosen, preface, viii.

[16]Sigmund Freud, "The Psychogenesis of a Case of Homosexuality in a Woman," Freud on Women: A Reader, ed. Elisabeth Young-Bruehl (New York: Norton, 1990) 241-266.

[17]Juliet Mitchell, Psychoanalysis and Feminism (New York: Vintage, 1974) 47.

[18]Victor J. Seidler, "Men, Sex and Relationships," Men, Sex and Relationships, ed. Seidler (London: Routledge, 1992) 5.

[19]Sigmund Freud, A Case of Hysteria, Three Essays on Sexuality and Other Works, vol. VII of The Complete Psychological Works (London: Hogarth, 1953, 1981).

[20]Jacqueline Rose, introduction-II, Feminine Sexuality: Jacques Lacan and the "école freudienne", ed. Juliet Mitchell and Rose (New York: Norton, 1982) 44.

[21]Mitchell, P & F, 107.

[22]Mitchell, P & F, 107.

[23]Mitchell, P & F, 53.

[24]Freud, Three Essays, 242.

[25]Helene Deutsch, "The Psychology of Women in Relation to the Functions of Reproduction (1924)," Women & Analysis: Dialogues on Psychoanalytic Views of Femininity, ed. Jean Strouse (Boston: G. K. Hall, 1985)150.

[26]Luce Irigaray, This Sex Which is Not One, trans. Catherine Porter (Ithaca: Cornell UP, 1977, 1985) 28.

[27]Irigaray 28.

[28]Karen Horney, "The Flight from Womanhood: The Masculinity-Complex in Women as Viewed by Men and by Women (1926)," Women & Analysis: Dialogues on Psychoanalytic Views of Femininity, ed. Jean Strouse (Boston: G. K. Hall, 1985) 184.

[29]Judith Kestenberg, "Outside and Inside, Male and Female," The Journal of the American Psychoanalytic Association 16 (1968) 507-508.

[31]Nancy Chodorow, The Reproduction of Mothering (Berkeley: U of California P, 1978) 166.

[32]Chodorow 167.

[33]Chodorow 176.

[34]Mitchell, P & F, 71.

[35]Irigary 39.

[36]John Brenkman, Straight Male Modern: A Cultural Critique of Psychoanalysis (New York: Routledge, 1993) 8-9.

[37]Juliet Mitchell, "On Freud and the Distinction Between the Sexes," Women & Analysis: Dialogues on Psychoanalytic Views of Femininity, ed. Jean Strouse (Boston: G. K. Hall, 1985) 34.

[38]Chodorow 181.

[39]Gerda Siann, Gender, Sex and Sexuality: Contemporary Psychological Perspectives (London: Taylor & Francis, 1994) 132-142.

[39]Susan Faludi, Backlash: The Undeclared War Against Women (London: Vintage, 1992).

[40]Joseph Pleck, The Myth of Masculinity (Cambridge: MIT P, 1981) 96.

[41]Thomas 14.

[42]Thomas 46.

[43]Thomas 191.

[44]Thomas 31.

[45]Brenkman 59.

[46]Brenkman 237.

[47]Brenkman 237.

[48]Brenkman 239.

[49]Brenkman 238.

[50]Rose 33.

[51]Jacques Lacan, The Four Fundamental Concepts of Psycho-Analysis, trans. Alan Sheridan (New York: Norton, 1981) 204.

[52]Lacan, FFC, 204.

[53]Lacan, FFC, 204.

[54]Jacques Lacan, Ecrits, trans. Alan Sheridan (New York: Norton, 1977) 285.

[55]Lacan, Ecrits, 285.

[56]Lacan, Ecrits, 287.

[57]Lacan, Ecrits, 18.

[58]Lacan, Ecrits, 19.

[59]Lacan, Ecrits, 19.

[60]Lacan, Ecrits, 4.

[61]Jonathan Scott Lee, Jacques Lacan (Amherst: U of Mass P, 1990) 20.

[62]Lee 59.

[63]Lacan, Ecrits, 263.

[64]Lacan, FFC, 235.

[65]Lee 66.

[66]Rose 42.

[67]Juliet Mitchell, introduction-I, Feminine Sexuality: Jacques Lacan and the "école freudienne", ed. Mitchell and Jacqueline Rose (New York: Norton, 1982) 19.

[68]Mark Bracher, Lacan, Discourse, and Social Change: A Psychoanalytic Cultural Criticism (Ithaca: Cornell UP, 1993) 34.

[69]Slavoj Zizek, The Sublime Object of Ideology (London: Verso, 1989) 118.

[70]Bracher 19.

[71]Kaja Silverman, Male Subjectivity at the Margins (New York: Routledge, 1992) 6.

[72]Silverman 15.

[73]Thomas 17.

CHAPTER III

THE EIGHTEENTH CENTURY'S REGENDERED MAN

From the moment I could talk, I was ordered to listen.

Cat Stevens, "Father and Son"[1]

Scholars as diverse as Michael McKeon, Thomas Laqueur, Michel Foucault, Lawrence Stone, Eve Kosofsky Sedgwick, Jeffrey Weeks, Nancy Armstrong, and Terry Eagleton have all recognized a shift in human sexual relations during the late-seventeenth and the eighteenth centuries.[2] This shift emphasizes fundamental differences, and what emerges from the discourse of that time is a "persuasive opinion . . . that each sex had its own modes of expression and its own separate sources of authority."[3] At first glance, this new perspective can be seen as a triumph for a resilient male authority,[4] but the epistemology that determines difference also questions it, and what results from this emphasis on establishing discernible sex roles is a great deal of eighteenth century discourse which discusses how men and women should behave. We are, ourselves, a product of this discourse and our continued efforts to expose the cultural facades placed over sexuality indicate the failure of that epistemology to coherently classify the difference. The persistence, for example, of the feminist voice, which began as a part of this eighteenth century discourse in the writings of women such as Mary Astell, Aphra Behn, and Mary Wollstonecraft, indicates the resistance and refusal of individuals to accept the gender roles predominant in their culture.

Usually, an examination of the new gender roles which develop during the eighteenth century has focused on the female and her increasingly restricted role in the family and home as well as her role as writer and often dissident voice.[5] My aim is to turn our gaze for the moment on the man, whose own gender position can also be assumed to have changed during this shift of human sexual relations. The work of Weeks, Randolph Trumbach, and Alan Bray has demonstrated that the status of "homosexual male" was, in a sense, institutionalized by increased legal attention and social isolation in the late-seventeenth and eighteenth centuries,[6] but little discussion has taken place about the heterosexual male except in conjunction with his oppositional position of power in relation to the female and homosexual male. By turning our gaze on the male, we break from a tradition that has assumed the consistency of his sexuality, and by penetrating his fictions of manhood, we expose the incompleteness and anxiety which "lies" beneath the surface of his seemingly secure identities. Any dramatic alterations to sexual relations which occurred in and around the eighteenth century must have been affected by and affected male subjectivity. The bigger questions are in what way did the male role change and why did those changes take place?

Discussions of male images like the capitalist, the imperialist, or the head of the household, which are generally viewed as roles which men desire to be, do not allow for the uneven interest that men have shown in embodying these images. Viewing male sexuality as unproblematic ignores the complexity of male desires and the variety of manly behaviors, some which coincide with culturally accepted manliness and some which avoid the cultural definition. Looking at man as monolith denies his lived experience as an often inconsequential body with a variety of prohibited desires and overlooks his numerous attempts to often transgressively reformulate his image in the persona of a rogue, a pirate, a gunfighter, or a member of a street gang. Our gaze must penetrate man's engendered image and reveal those desires which move him toward both the socially acceptable and the socially intolerable. Accordingly, as Lyndal Roper has said, "if gender is to be a category of social explanation, it must bridge the gap between discourse, social formation and the individual sexed subject."[7] This bridge is not easily constructed. The individual is always something more than discourse and something other than her or his social assignment. Yet, subjectivity can be analyzed only with the evidence available through discourse and social interaction and a look at the gender changes of the eighteenth century must begin with the evidence at hand.

According to Foucault, during the eighteenth century "things went from ritual lamenting over the unfruitful debauchery of the rich, bachelors, and libertines to a discourse in which the sexual conduct of the population was taken both as an object of analysis and as a target of intervention."[8] Retrospectively, this "project" to restrict sexual conduct can be seen (as Foucault sees it) as "not succeeding" and instead causing an "age of multiplication: a dispersion of sexualities, a strengthening of their disparate forms, a multiple implantation of 'perversions',"[9] and the development of these sexualities can be seen as part of an effort to create an order of sexual conduct which privileges certain behaviors while chastising, shunning, or punishing others. Roy Porter has argued that whereas Enlightenment England experienced an increased interest in and discussion of sex and "reconceptualised sexuality as being an essential part of Nature," by the end of the eighteenth century, "[10]Bowdlerism, Grundyism, prudery, repression, anxiety and shame were summoned up to put sexuality back in its rightful place."[11] In Eric Trudgill's words, "Society had in fact throughout the century become progressively more decorous in its [sexual] manners,"[12] a change he attributes to the influence of "middle-class sexual attitudes" and a "pious and moral throne," but, most importantly, to the "gradual acceptance of the idea that flagrant vice was a sign of inferior taste."[13] In effect, a sexual hierarchy was being created which assigned significant social values to various sexual roles.

During the eighteenth century, a discursive preoccupation with sex, or, in Foucault's words, a "political, economic, and technical incitement to talk about sex,"[14] intensified in an apparent effort to set boundaries between and among the sexes. Seemingly, most of this discourse was directed at females. In "countless conduct books and works of instruction,"[15] according to Nancy Armstrong, writers repeatedly focused on the female in their efforts to describe behaviors which would make women more suitable counterparts as daughters and wives to men. Through the novel, as Armstrong has also pointed out, woman became the model of morality and domesticity in support of the new economic man.[16] Even in empirical discussions, as Laqueur has shown, the focus of difference was placed on the woman whose "problematic, unstable" body was compared to "the unproblematic, stable male body."[17] Laqueur further theorizes that changes in epistemology caused a shift in how the body was viewed anatomically: a one body anatomical system which presupposed the female body as a lesser version of the male was replaced by a two body system which searched for fundamental differences between the sexes. In the latter system, however, the male body remained the physiological standard while the female body became the object of analysis and speculation.[18]

In an age known for increasing skepticism, questions regarding the female body, female sexuality, and innate female virtue are not surprising. What should strike us is the nonchalance with which the male body and male sexuality went unobserved and unquestioned. Gender roles are fostered in a community of interconnected sexed subjects, and members of both sexes contribute to, take part in, and suffer from the engendering process. While the new role of woman expected her to deny her desires and led to, according to Foucault, "an hysteriza-tion of women's bodies,"[19] the manner in which man was allowed to enact his desires was also restricted: on the one hand sublimating sexual desire into production while, on the other hand, repressing desire only to have it appear in a variety of "perversions" such as voyeurism, exhibitionism, necrophilia, sadism, and masochism.[20]

What changed in the manner in which males and females identi-fied themselves as men and women is especially important when considering what did not change. Instead of creating a more reason-able and equitable relation between the sexes, new gender roles promoted male authority and female subordination in a continuation of patriarchal power which contradicted the other political and economic developments of the time. A society characterized by an epistemology which encouraged individualism, democratic princi-ples, a free market economy, and a mobile class system[21] paradoxi-cally supported a hierarchical division of the sexes and a restriction of female subjectivity. At the same time that political, economic, and social power was separated from patrilineage, that same power was interwoven with gender roles.

This perpetuation and, in some cases, intensification of differ-ences between the genders[22] has proven to be an always uncertain and generally impossible project primarily because both sexes inconveniently fail to fit into their exclusive gender roles. Females have found these roles in the "modern system of gender difference"[23] especially limiting and it is no coincidence that historically feminism found its strongest early voice at the end of the eighteenth century in

Wollstonecraft.[24] Males, on the other hand, have seldom questioned this system, perhaps because it provides a control of females for which most males are willing to repress all but culturally accepted desires. This repression, however, has its consequences in the form of neurotic symptoms and perverse behavior. Male silence, while arguably part of the gender role of man, may also indicate a strong psychic defense against male desire. On a cultural level, the major restructuring of gender, in spite of this conflict with individual desire, suggests a strong resistance to change from the earlier patriarchal structure. Rather than question the male body and, by extension, its preeminence, the growing field of medical science chose instead to focus on the female's differences. Because of this omission of an examination of the male anatomy, Laqueur has said that "it is probably not possible to write a history of man's body and its pleasures because the historical record was created in a cultural tradition where no such history was necessary."[25] Significantly, the new epistemology, with all of its skepticism, would continue to avoid questions about the male body and about the foundation of masculinity and male power.

This impetus to establish gender boundaries which identify "woman" as sexual object conceals an uncertain basis for the newly gendered "man". If "woman" becomes gendered as the spectacle and "man" as the spectator during the eighteenth century, which Armstrong[26] and Kristina Straub,[27] among others, contend, then woman's construction as the object of the gaze coincides with a turn of the gaze away from the culturally-redefined "man". Traditionally, a look at 'man' has been a peripheral glance which assumes that he is complete and in control of the world he has constructed. He is, for example, man the warrior, man the architect, or man the business tycoon. However, if we look closer, the lives and desires of males generally fail to live up to the expectations of their gender position. Paradoxically, just like the differences between men and women, these demands of manhood become important at a time when the political and social hierarchy is being dismantled.

The increased emphasis on female conduct and heightened interest in the female anatomy as well as an attempt to "establish a differential masculine standard of value"[28] coincides with what McKeon argues (following Laqueur) is a change of perspective when an "ontological" view of sex replaces a "sociological" one,[29] at a time when a "regime of difference" historically replaces a "regime of hierarchy."[30] In other words, the epistemological changes which occurred during the Restoration and the eighteenth century restructured patriarchy by disassociating power from aristocratic birth and then connecting that power with presumably natural superior qualities. Women, in this view, are inferior to men by nature and, subsequently, should be educated in such a way so that they can occupy themselves with tasks which fit their character.[31] Differences between males, however, can chiefly be demonstrated by relating the male to the female, which is done in the creation of types such as "Gentleman," "Pretty Fellow," "Coxcomb," "Rake," or "Fop,"[32] or by citing personal accomplishments. However, what constitutes success is never easily defined, and the changing economic, political, and social environment of late-seventeenth-century and eighteenth-century Britain made proving manhood an ominous project. Without the hierarchical rules contingent upon hereditary authority, the question of what makes one man different from the next is extremely difficult to answer.

Male subjectivity, in this environment, can be seen as a balancing act that was constantly requiring adjustment to the conditions which surrounded it, and those conditions were constantly changing because of their inability to satisfy male subjects, or, in other words, to firmly establish what a "man" should be. Robert Markley, in describing the seventeenth-century physico-theologian Robert Boyle's use of the word "gentleman" states:

> a "gentleman" is not simply a social given but also an unstable entity that must be continually redefined and reinscribed to present the complexities, uncertainties, and ambiguities of social relations as a convenient--and simplified--opposition between "us" and "them"; in turn, the privileged term of this binary construction, the gentleman, contains unending social and economic negotiations to determine (always contingent) hierarchical positions of rank, stature, and power.[33]

The male instability that Markley describes results not only from an individual opportunity to move up or down in the hierarchy, but also from the instability of the hierarchy itself. Once all men have access to the same resources and can assume the same expectations, then all men are prey to each other's judgment. In fact, those subjective judgments construct the hierarchy's structure by either supporting or denying each male's right to call himself a man (or, in Markley's example, a gentleman) and to assume the power assigned to that role. A successful man has certain social skills, possesses certain material goods, and establishes his family in a certain manner, and, subsequently, this man can expect to be viewed by others in a certain way. Of course, what qualifies as the appropriate skills, goods, and family are subject to frequent revision since the other's perspective is never fixed. In the eighteenth century, therefore, defining the better man, or the gentleman, became complex, problematic, and the potential cause of masculine anxiety since hereditary authority no longer provided the definition.

The masculine gender role of economic or "Public man"[34] which emerges from the eighteenth century ruled the world of commerce outside the home, but this man no longer possessed the security of unquestioned patriarchal power. Once Enlightenment thought became engaged in an epistemology which centered knowledge and understanding within the individual, patriarchal authority was dead, and the power or lack of power which each person derived from that authority was open to question. As historian Christopher Hill points out, the execution of Charles I prompted an examination of all authority. "All traditional institutions were called in question, including the Bible, private property, marriage and the family, [and] male superiority,"[35] but these examinations were prohibited once power fell into the hands of a group of "business men" whose "main concern" was "to preserve property and social subordination."[36] On a political level, the role of Parliament in making laws and in governing the country survived the questioning of its authority and largely changed only in its relationship to the king; it retained and even increased its power to alter the lives of the citizenry. On a domestic level, the father maintained his power over the household, and an expanding variety of economic opportunities became available to men. Nevertheless, beneath this maintenance of male power positions, the questions regarding the advantages given to some and not others remained unanswered. In the absence of the king and his authority, everyone has a potentially equal right to pursue pleasure, and all positions of power, including those which are connected to just being a man, seem arbitrary and suspect.

When Charles I's head fell on January 30, 1649, the absolute power of the English monarchy symbolically ended. At the moment the King's head was separated from his body, a type of order and security were irretrievably lost. As the historical presence of the Restoration indicates, attempts would be made to put things back where they were, but the regicides had made their point: a king could be judged by his subjects and his blood was not sacred.[37] Nevertheless, after the Restoration, many of the surviving regicides and the disinterred corpses of those, like Oliver Cromwell, who had not survived were themselves beheaded. The symbolic nature of their punishment not only mirrors the King's fate but also duplicates the "un-manning" action of the execution. Just as the King's authority had been symbolically severed, so had the authority of those who had assumed his power. Subsequently, this power would belong to the propertied class, many of whom had supported both the elimination of the sovereign and the retributive punishment against the King's executioners. "The gentry and merchant oligarchies,"[38] whose primary agenda promoted political stability and economic growth, would thereafter work toward a compromise between absolute authority and radical republicanism. This compromise was characterized by what Hill terms the Hanoverian Settlement of 1689, which placed the importance of patrilineal descent beneath the economic, political and religious needs and purposes of the property owners. In effect, patriarchal sovereignty had been castrated and a consensual government would be erected in its place.

An insight into the psychical consequences of this loss of sovereignty can be gained by examining Freud's Totem and Taboo, in which he describes the mythical killing of the first sovereign, the primal father, by a union of brothers who unite to acquire the father's sexual dominion. In Freud's description of the primal horde, the brothers unite to kill the father and acquire sexual access to the women that have been denied to them, but when the father is dead, their ambivalent feelings of love and hate toward him cause them guilt and their fear of rivalry causes them to renounce their claims to the women. In "deferred obedience"[39] to the father, the brothers establish a "father-surrogate"[40] in the form of a totem which also represents their longing for the father, a reminder of their filial pact, and the source of their power. "Nevertheless," Freud states, "it would be a mistake to suppose that the hostile impulses inherent in the father-complex were completely silenced during this period of revived paternal authority."[41] The ambivalent attitude of the brothers toward the father remains as well as the repressed desires which caused both his murder and resurrection in the form of a totem.

Freud's narrative outlines the dual nature of the brother's psychical condition before and after the father's murder:

Before	After
1. Desire to be rid of the father	1. Longing for the father
2. Sexual desire	2. Sexual denial
3. Fear of the father	3. Fear of each other
4. Desire for power	4. Desire for restraint
5. Women elevated as objects of desire	5. Women cast out as a source of division and as a reminder of guilt

The chronological sequence of these psychical states should not be seen as the later conditions superseding the former; rather, both states continue to exist simultaneously and in obvious conflict.

Transposition of Freud's mythological narrative with the complex events of history would be a misleading rhetorical maneuver, but the psychical consequences of this mythical filial power struggle provide a valuable insight into the actual struggle for power which followed the execution of the King. Carole Pateman has observed how men abandoned the patriarchy at this time for a brotherhood which, in effect, handed patriarchal power from the father to the fraternity of brothers.[42] In Pateman's analysis, "Modern patriarchy is fraternal in form and the original [sexual] contract is a fraternal pact,"[43] and

"Freud's conjectural history of the origin of social life,"[44] follows a pattern similar to the historical movement from paternal rule to civil society. Likewise, Eve Kosofsky Sedgwick has discussed how men during the late seventeenth and eighteenth century developed methods of homosocial behavior in an effort to establish and maintain relations with other men.[45] Both Pateman and Sedgwick point out the importance of the subordination of women in these negotiations between men; however, the negotiations take place because the men fear each other and desire to find a means of mutual restraint upon which they can all agree. While the threat of female authority, as Pateman argues, was a possibility (at least, psychically), the most immediate dangers posed to men during this restructuring of power came from other men.

After the death of the primal father, like after the death of the King, people are returned to what John Locke in his defense of the Glorious Revolution called "the state of nature" where natural laws operate and each person is born with an executive power,[46] but people give up this power to the commonwealth, according to Locke, primarily because they wish to enjoy their property in "peace and safety," or, in other words, they want to protect their "life, liberty, and estate" from each other.[47] A key to Locke's argument, as Linda J. Nicholson points out, is his "separation of the familial and the political," which provides men a natural power in the limited sphere of the nuclear family while claiming that the power of kings was unnatural and different in kind from that of fathers.[48] At the same time that he promotes the unity of family, as Nicholson also notes, Locke denies the greater kinship relations available through other possible relationships between and among women and men.[49] In terms analogous to Freud's myth, Locke suggests that the best way for the brothers to get along is to deny the father, divide the women, and make a pact which will guarantee mutual security.

However, the ambivalent attitude of the mythical brothers toward the father, their simultaneous love and hate and their guilt and desire, is reflected in the actual historical events and the discourse which followed the dissolution of absolutism. The government that was formed can be viewed as an uneasy compromise between a desire to take power from the king and a desire to return the king to his absolutist patriarchal throne. Edmund Burke, defending that Government of compromise more than one hundred years after Locke, wrote:

> Government is a contrivance of human wisdom to provide for human <u>wants</u>. Men have a right that these wants should be provided for by this wisdom. Among these wants is to be reckoned the want, out of civil society, of a sufficient restraint upon their passions. . . . This can only be done <u>by a power out of themselves</u>; and not, in the exercise of its function, subject to that will and to those passions which it is its office to bridle and subdue.[50] [Burke's emphasis]

In Burke's view, the government is a necessary fiction, a "contrivance," that restrains individual passions for the sake of civility. Behind this view is his fear of a repetition in England of the violent events in France which he also compares to "a Revolution which happened in England."[51] Burke's comments are particularly revealing because they reflect the before and after motivations of the confederation of brothers: individual passions and a fear of those passions. Burke believes that men need to agree upon a government or law which, like the mythical totem, assumes and symbolizes patriarchal authority and enforces the restraint of each other's desires.

Like the mythical brothers, Burke also longs for the father, or a return to the day when the King's authority kept everyone under control. In his words, "The age of chivalry is gone. That of sophisters, economists, and calculators, has succeeded; and the glory of Europe is extinguished for ever."[52] Yet, he is not a proponent of a return to absolutism but an advocate of compromise. Power belongs neither to one man nor to all men, but to an independent entity which somehow possesses a wisdom lacking in the individual. "It is therefore of infinite importance that [people at large] should not be suffered to imagine that their will, any more than that of kings, is the standard of right and wrong."[53] The government, in Burke's view, should provide that standard. The "new intellectual syntheses of John Locke and Isaac Newton"[54] demanded reasons to support a hierarchical order and Burke, as an inheritor of Enlightenment thought, is more interested in reasoning against the anarchy he sees in France and fears in England than attempting to justify a new hierarchical alignment. Instead, he proposes a seemingly neutral outside "contrivance," the government, to keep everyone in order.

The conditions that Burke describes surrounding the creation of the new English Government after the death of the King are similar to the events which develop with the primal horde after the father's murder. Killing a king, or, more exactly, epistemologically removing his symbolic basis of power, challenges all phallic authority. In the absence of the King, a great deal of discourse was generated to justify maintaining patriarchal power and to establish a new division of that power. A government would eventually be formed which would attempt to balance both the need for a phallic presence and continued patriarchal control with the growing importance of the individual and his subjective power. In other words, the longing for a sovereign remained in spite of the contradictory desire for self-rule. This political ambiguity mirrors the brothers' ambivalent feelings toward the father in Freud's narrative, where love and admiration exist in conflict with fear and desire. Psychically, the desire to remove a king with all of its corresponding fears remains antagonistically in concert with a longing for a king with all of its attendant passions. The pact which replaces the king parallels the covenant which binds the brothers in the absence of the father, and though this historical pact is called the Law or the Government, it resembles the mythical totem which the brothers use to represent the dead father as well as their fraternal agreement and to symbolize and provide the phallic authority which they now inherit.

In order to understand the impact of these political changes on the individual male, it is important to recognize the unsettling nature of this epistemological shift. As Locke's arguments about civil government indicate, the dissolution of the King's absolute authority had potential ramifications for all kinship relations. Only by distinguishing a father's power from a king's can Locke propose the maintenance of the family at the same time that he argues for a government without a patriarchal head. Locke retains the father's power by locating the family ahistorically[55] and relying on biology to support his contention that the father is a natural protector while a king is not. This separation of familial and political power allows Locke, like the later Burke, to retain a traditionally male authority while recognizing the deficiencies of a patriarchical political system. What both Locke and Burke argue against, however, is the loss of structure which they view as coincidental to a loss of control over the passions of others. Locke differentiates between "the dissolution of the society and the dissolution of the government,"[56] and says that "no man in civil society can be exempted from the laws of it."[57] Burke acknowledges human desires, or "wants," but sees government as a necessary check on those desires. Both writers recognize a conflict between individual desires and societal needs, and both assert that consent among individuals is the basis for restrictions on desire; however, both argue defensively in fear of the anarchy which they imply would result from the loss of paternal authority (Locke) or the absence of a superior power which can hold desires in check (Burke). In either case, the role of the male shifts from one of hierarchical certainty to one of societal complicity. The essence of this masculine role, however, contains a built-in anxiety caused by the gap between the newly developing male authority and its separation from the original source of male power, the King, or as Sir Robert Filmer argued in <u>Patriarcha</u>, Adam.[58]

The consequences to male subjectivity caused by a realignment of patriarchal authority can be better understood by examining these political and social changes in Lacanian structural terms. In Lacan's view, the Freudian myth of the primal horde operates on the imaginary and symbolic levels,[59] and the totem erected in the Name-of-the-Father can be seen as representing the phallus, a signifier which, in the absence of the father, anchors the Law of the Father in language. "The phallus," according to Lacan, "is not a phantasy, if by that we mean an imaginary effect. Nor is it as such an object (part-, internal, good, bad, etc.) in the sense that this term tends to accentuate the reality pertaining in a relation. It is even less the organ, penis or clitoris, that it symbolizes."[60] Instead, the phallus represents an attempt to resist symbolically the fundamental lack-of-being that an individual psychically experiences and is used to establish a chain of signifiers which provide a meaning for existence. Similarly, on a cultural level, the phallus represents (in its absence) the source of structure for kinship relations and, consequently, the power relations between genders. In the eighteenth century, the pact between men which Locke and Burke describe relocates the phallic power of a king in the civil institutions of society while restructuring gender relations (incorporating the nuclear family) to adapt to this revised patriarchal authority.

Nevertheless, there is a gap within the structure of the phallus which makes phallic power illusory. At the same time the phallus is used to provide meaning through metonymically-linked chains of signifiers, it resists signification and is, in Lacan's words, "the signifier for which there is no signified."[61] All meaning structured on the phallus, therefore, is attached ultimately to that which cannot be expressed. Consequently, on the one hand, the phallus represents that which exists outside of language: a totality of meaning, generative power, unrestricted pleasure, and immortality; however, on the other hand, the phallus is an illusion, a void located at the center of language. Absolutism, for example, corresponded to a need to see a human embodiment of the phallus and dissolved when this mirage could no longer be reasonably believed. Once the phallus is called into question, however, the phallic law which politically and socially privileges certain men is also suspect. Consequently, in the late seventeenth and eighteenth century the relationship of the male to symbolic possession of the phallus, or manhood, moves from the assurance of phallic authority symbolically embodied by a king to a condition of phallic uncertainty where manhood is always on trial. Male subjectivity, therefore, becomes a matter of proving possession of a power associated with the phallus, and the best way to offer that proof is to differentiate masculinity from the otherness of femininity and to distinguish one form of manhood from others.

If a male is to be identified as a man he must be linked to and seemingly shown to have the phallus,[62] but this is problematic because of the illusory nature of the phallus and because of the fluxional character of those signifiers which allow the individual to stake a claim to the phallus. In other words, certain signifiers generally associated with "man" like "strong", "brave", "hard-working", and "virile" are open to both individual and cultural interpretation and qualification; subsequently, being a man means undertaking the tenuous task of physically and symbolically embodying an unstable set of signifiers. In the eighteenth century, a number of significant cultural changes take place which suggest an attempt to anchor manhood by defining it with new terms tied to the changing cultural environment. Much of the discourse of this period, especially the discourse regarding sex, results as a defensive maneuvering in response to attacks on established masculine positions.

Between men, differences in birthright were gradually being replaced by economic differences evident in the initial stages of development of a class structure,[63] the genesis of professions, most notably at the lower levels of the medical and legal professions,[64] and the beginnings of an institutionalization of poverty as new social concern and philanthropy gave rise to what would become the modern welfare state.[65] Notably, even as heredity became a suspect basis for power, gender differences continued to decide who could have political, economic, and social control and differences between men came to be defined increasingly by the nature and level of power that a male possessed.

The re-gendering of individuals during the eighteenth century occurs as part of the restructuring of these on-going patriarchal divisions. A growing amount of discourse about female chastity and an increased anxiety about male homosexuality more and more relegated the woman to the home and domestic matters and created, through alienation and persecution, a homosexual community.[66] This emphasis on the sexual behavior of women and gay men underscores the insecurity of the patriarchal system and the power it provides to heterosexual men. By discussing woman, eighteenth century commentators avoided discussing man and confronting the myth of male superiority. Through strengthened prohibitions against male homosexuality (but significantly, not against female homosexuality[67]) male sexuality was defined not only through difference to female sexuality but in strict denial of any desires which might be considered feminine. Rather than examining the fragile foundation of male power, most discourse looked away from the phallus and toward those individuals who could clearly be denied phallic authority.

Discourse focused on the woman and the gay man avoids acknowledging that no one possesses the phallus and that males, though they have a penis and a mythical connection to the phallus, are, in reality, as castrated as females, having no claim to the immortality and omnipotence that phallic power includes. In this way, male subjectivity is a defensive project based upon an illusion of phallic significance, "a kind of collective make-believe in the commensurability of penis and phallus,"[68] according to Kaja Silverman, which is realized by pretending that man is complete and empowered. One way to place the male in this phallic gender position is to situate what constitutes "man" in opposition to what constitutes a symbolically castrated "woman". Rather than proving man to be worthy of his position of authority, it is easier to prove woman unworthy. If, as Susan Dwyer Amussen has said, during the eighteenth century "the subordination of women was far more important to men than to women,"[69] it is because a stable identity for woman was made more necessary because of the male's insecure position as man. Consequently, even as technology during the eighteenth century diminished the importance of the male's "degree of physical superiority,"[70] his only advantage according to Wollstonecraft, feminine weakness became more important as a metaphor for a number of deficiencies of mind, body, and character assigned to the female in her role as woman.

On the one hand, therefore, "woman" is a convenient fiction, an other who in her limited condition supports male authority by her incapacity. On the other hand, however, "woman" also represents a diversion, a temporary escape, from male/male power relations. In this sense, she acts as a mode of exchange between men, a point emphasized in Sedgwick's work. In an effort to develop same-sex social bonds, according to Sedgwick, men in the eighteenth century intensified their employment of the female as a third term. Using a woman as the conduit for their desire, men could compete or unite with other men based upon their relationship with a woman or women. This legitimized "homosocial" behavior allows male desire for other men to get played out in a socially accepted arena while reinforcing a heterosexual doctrine and the homophobia that accompanies that doctrine. "Women," Sedgwick notes in her examination of Shakespeare's sonnets, "are merely the vehicles by which men breed more men, for the gratification of other men."[71] In this way, women become a tool for male stratification. Sedgwick demonstrates how male bonding can occur through cuckoldry, the sexual sharing of a woman, in William Wycherly's The Country Wife, but more often a woman is portrayed as the site of a male power struggle which the best man wins (as in Tom Jones where Tom proves himself the "naturally" better man and wins Sophia from Mr. Blifil). With women gaining more choice in their marriage partners during the century, the reality of male confrontations over a female grows and becomes a common theme in the development of the novel. Even in a heroine-centered novel like Fanny Burney's Evelina, the superior masculinity of Lord Orville is described in contrast to other male characters like the dishonorable, deceitful Sir Clement Willoughby, the "weak and evasive"[72] M. DuBois, the rowdy Mr. Coverly, the immature Mr. Broughton, the profligate Lord Merton, and the foppish Mr. Lovel.

Woman, then, is one standard against which men may measure themselves, and, like most standards of measurement, she is most useful when she returns the same readings every time. By targeting women readers, by encouraging specific female attributes, and by creating a discourse for, about, and often by women, writers separated the expected experience of the female from the male's political world, but, at the same time, these same writers established a world where woman had their own form of power. As Nancy Armstrong states:

> Literature devoted to producing the domestic woman thus appeared to ignore the political world run by men. Of the female alone did it presume to say that neither birth nor the accoutrements of title and status accurately represented the individual; only the more subtle nuances of behavior indicated what one was really worth.[73]

In Armstrong's opinion, women acquired an individuality that men did not, but the more clearly the characteristics of woman are defined, the more easily a man may avoid adopting those characteristics. For example, Armstrong and others have claimed that emotional qualities became a part of the feminine sphere[74] during this time period. According to Terry Eagleton, women became "canonized" in their "role as specialists in sentiment."[75] Yet, when women are made the masters of emotion, men are simultaneously being signaled to be unemotional. If the signifier "woman" is important as a category (and the quantity of discourse demonstrates the importance of this signifier), then those signifiers which indicate "woman-ness" are metonymically important. Being a "man" means not being a "woman" and not possessing womanly characteristics. So, instead of seeing the new domestic woman as Armstrong does, "a woman whose value resided chiefly in her femaleness . . ., one who, in other words, excelled in the qualities that differentiated her from the male,"[76] the domestic woman can be viewed as a useful aggregation of characteristics that the new economic man was supposed to avoid.

This reinforced emphasis on non-feminine male conduct is illustrated in the increasingly oppressive treatment of male homosexuals during this same time period. Alan Bray, in <u>Homosexuality in Renaissance England,</u> notes that some time around the Restoration homophobia became institutionalized and gay males began their own subculture.[77] Coincidental with this segregation of gay males was the (often erroneous) association of feminine qualities with men who engaged in homosexual relationships. Prior to this time, as McKeon points out, male homosexuality was seen as an aberration, but such relationships did not infringe upon masculinity.[78] Eventually, however, gay males were ostracized and stereotyped as womanly or effeminate, a word itself which McKeon shows gradually took on a more restricted and negative meaning. In terms of the sexual hierarchy, therefore, men desiring homosexual relationships could keep these relationships private or fall out of the male political sphere. The creation of a separate subculture became a necessity. Additionally, these males had almost no social value since, unlike women, they served no clear function in the advancement of the patriarchal agenda.

This does not mean that the creation of the womanly molly served no purpose. On the contrary, this image secures masculinity by identifying the pitfalls of its opposite, femininity. The need to define manhood required an example of forfeited masculinity. Female traits cannot be discouraged in men if an example of what happens to those who acquire these traits does not exist. The creation of the modern male homosexual stereotype, therefore, reinforced the heterosexual male's position as not-female while establishing for homosexual males a political class, albeit an excluded and persecuted class. Male desire became strictly defined as male heterosexual desire.

Like women, therefore, homosexual men gained a special significance during the eighteenth century as part of an effort to define masculinity and secure male power within those masculine boundaries. Subsequently, the heterosexual male was privileged because of the presence of male genitalia and the rejection of female qualities. Nevertheless, this privilege with its clearly sexual connections becomes problematic when heterosexual males are evaluated against each other. As stated above, possession of the correct woman or women provides one source of proof of sexual superiority, but to the new economic man she represents just one commodity that satisfies the demands of manhood. In a world where men were no longer as economically restricted by birth as in the past and could aspire to a higher status, the acquisition of property, real and personal, became a prominent means of demonstrating superior masculinity.

Eagleton argues that the project to create woman was joined by a project to create a new middle class man with the anti-aristocratic (others might read these as Protestant) "values of thrift, peace and chastity."79 While writers promoted these values, however, men do not appear to have accepted them as a part of their sexuality. Eagleton's contention that "the barbarous values of militarism, naked dominance and male hauteur, badges of predatory public aristocracy, [were] mollified by the fashionable virtues of uxoriousness, sensibility, civility and tendresse"80 would seem overstated, or at least short-lived, in view of the displays of male power that dominate the nineteenth and twentieth centuries. If a permanent "mollification" (an interesting term in view of the development of a gay male sub-culture at this time) of male aggression did occur, it was a cosmetic alteration made necessary by a growing economic reliance on trade. For, although the manners of the social male were modeled on gentility, a quality previously assumed in possession of the nobility but extended to those who were newly acquiring wealth and property,[81] the male objective remained hierarchical. Masculinity was evidenced by the standards of wealth, power, and status, and though civility was a nice quality, power was a more important instrument in the fulfillment of desires. As much as commentators might wish to plead the contrary, the kindest, most noble beggar did not have the sexual presence of the rudest, most vulgar Lord.

Of course, the idea of a sexual presence is problematic because of the subjective nature of sexuality, but no one can dispute that the satisfaction of sexual desire seems more available to men with power than to men without. What complicates this rather simple equation of power = satisfaction is that the nature of desire always means that the object of desire (the object $\underline{a}$ or missing object signified by the phallus) is psychically unobtainable. Every attempt at fulfillment is accompanied by a feeling that something has been left out. While a male may be defined by others as a man because of his accomplishments, intellect, skills, or financial capabilities, he remains fundamentally unsatisfied and unable to rest assured of a masculinity dependent upon the opinion of others. The image of the phallus, a monolithic symbol of generative power complete in itself, represents the impossible standard against which the male judges himself. The dissolution of absolutism removed phallic authority since a king and his lineage was the embodiment of the phallus, but the hierarchy that remained still utilized this myth to maintain power. The new epistemology had symbollically castrated the King, and, in doing so, had both opened the doors to power for other men and simultaneously made all claims to sovereignty suspect. In other words, on an individual level, each man was faced with proving his manhood, his connection to the phallus, while knowing, often subconsciously, that this manhood was a facade. What followed, historically, was an intensi-fied attempt to define masculinity through others. This effort would fail, but not without solidifying the social divisions which continue to exist today.

Male subjectivity, therefore, can be seen as the donning of identi-ties which are recognized as related to the phallus; however, it can also be viewed as the result of an identification process that subli-mates desire into patterns which agree with acceptable male roles (the new economic man) and restricts the otherwise diverse sexual aims and objects of the body to those which have a clear connection to reproduction (compulsory heterosexuality). This latter attempt to fix the limits of acceptable sexual practices simultaneously defines and, in Foucault's opinion, creates perversions, or what Freud described as those "deviations in respect of the sexual aim"[82] that have no direct relationship with genital union for the purpose of procreation. When, as is generally the case, an individual's sexuality encompasses more than the desire to employ his or her body in this restrictive fashion, then that desire must be repressed (often only to return in neurotic symptoms), sublimated in a way which includes, for example, increased work effort and intellectual activity, or expressed in a manner classified as perverse by its exclusion from the definition of acceptable sexual behavior. During the eighteenth century, the increased attention paid to categorizing sexual behavior simultaneously heightened the possibility of repression, sublimation, and perversion. If the hysterical woman and the perverse adult were not created at this time, as Foucault claims they were,[83] this ex-panded interest in limiting sexual behavior fostered conditions which no doubt multiplied the opportunity for individuals to develop hysterical symptoms and participate in perverse behaviors. Likewise, however, males appear to have sublimated their desires in their work effort, subsequently producing an age of invention and expansion. In this environment, masculinity becomes a quest driven by sublimated desires toward a societally-sanctioned manly identity and away from those desires which have no place in a world governed more and more by the principles of utility.

While an historian like J. A. Sharpe no longer unquestionably accepts the convenient and traditional view of the eighteenth century as an age of industrialization and the growth of the middle class, a movement toward these cultural phenomena indisputably took place at this time. In addition, the eighteenth century marks the time when urbanization,[84] nationalism,[85] consumerism,[86] and professionalism[87] rapidly began to resemble their present-day appearance. These cultural trends share the characteristic of being simultaneously divisive and unifying, and each suggests the need for individuals to adopt identities (e.g., Londoner, Englishman, and Professor) which provide a differentiating value. Consequently, the result of these trends was, in Sharpe's words, a "steady increase in social stratification"[88] and a discourse which both justified and questioned the societal map which was being charted.

In terms of masculinity, this increase in social stratification created changing requirements for manhood while attempting to stabilize and secure the various strata of male identity. For example, the growing recognition of the medical, legal, and military professions during this time period can be seen as a result of both the improved (although uneven) performance of men in these occupations and the need to have men whom society believed could provide health, justice, or protection. With the establishment of a special niche created by public perception and need, men in each of these professions allied themselves to promote an image of authority and to defend against attacks and easy access by other men to this authority. Subsequently, entrance into these professions became increasingly restrictive.[89] In this instance, occupation provides a male with something extra that demonstrates masculinity, but men could be successful in other ways. Most obviously, a male who proves capable of obtaining, keeping, or displaying affluence exhibits a superior masculinity compared to the male with little money or possessions; however, less clearly, the male who violently controls others or who deceptively gets what he wants while others do not also exerts a masculine power. While the normative discourse of the eighteenth century promoted the first type of male struggle as economic competition, it denounced the second type as barbaric or criminal; nevertheless, both modes of masculinity share a demonstrated desire for authority and power over other men (and women). Inevitably, the difference between these two means to power must be indistinct.

In other words, in spite of all the discussions of morality which take place during the eighteenth century, masculinity remained dependent on the acquisition and retention of power. Males were confronted by an ever-changing terrain that required them to succeed in the city, under the increased scrutiny of others, and in the face of continued economic and technological developments. The epistemic shift (in Foucault's terms) that took place at this time both promoted the idea of a knowable universe while skeptically questioning every basis for knowledge, and it also encouraged colonial expansion, empirical investigation, and the growth of capital while wondering about the negative effects of progress. At a time when women were arguably being confined to the home, men were expected to compete and excel in this evolving world, but not all men were capable of succeeding in this changing environment. In fact, the majority of men may have become more powerless and more anonymous as the economy shifted away from self-employment to employment by others and as people moved into urban areas and away from the familiarity and recognizability of village life. In the past, a man had been most commonly identified by a role in the community that generally resembled his father's or that of another male relative or family acquaintance, but the changing economic landscape made these identities unstable and threatened a reassessment of each male's value. With the continued expansion of commerce, a previously unknown man, group of men, or technology could suddenly appear and not only challenge a man's trade but also impinge upon his position as a male. Those who prevailed in this struggle for male supremacy were installed as professionals and entrepreneurs, but those who failed had to search elsewhere for a male identity. As a result, masculinity for most men became narrowly defined by what they could control, their household position and their work effort.

However, these less empowered males did not necessarily lose their desire to express or display their masculinity. On an individual basis, each man deprived of societally-recognized power could accept some other social construct such as dominance over his wife, comradeship with his economic equals, or belief in his spiritual significance as proof of his male standing. Furthermore, he could always resist the powers that emasculated him by escaping into perversion, where he could play out his desires in an unlimited number of fantastic ways. The narrowing view of acceptable male sexual behavior not only encouraged men to sublimate their desires in an effort to rise in the male (sexual) hierarchy, but also pushed men inevitably toward sexual repression and symptomatic expression, and into their imaginations and toward perverse fantasy. Consequently, masculinity became an empirical quest which superseded rules and transcended boundaries, but always found itself short of the phallus and never regained even the mirage of absolute authority.

We can observe, for example, (as I do in the following chapter) the aggressive nature of the rake Lovelace in Samuel Richardson's Clarissa and the exemplary behavior of Richardson's "man of religion and virtue,"[90] Sir Charles Grandison, but we also need to understand why, at the end of the century, William Godwin could remark that "it would not perhaps be adventurous to affirm that more readers have wished to resemble Lovelace, than have wished to resemble Grandison."[91] Until his rape of Clarissa, Lovelace's ability to get all that he desires defines him as a male in possession of the phallus and makes him sexually attractive in a way which even his ultimate failure cannot erase. Male sexuality becomes not just a form of economic power, but is connected to the male's superiority to others, even if that superiority is defined by his transcendence of societal laws. Importantly, while the gender 'man' was being redefined during the eighteenth century, those anti-societal and aberrant characteristics which attracted readers to Lovelace and, later, to Gothic villains were also being incorporated into forms of masculinity.

The phallus exists outside of language and law, so unlawful behavior does not prevent and may even suggest that someone possesses phallic manhood. In our examination of the new gender identities being formed at this time, we need to be concerned with not only the types of men promoted and the desires discouraged by the discourse, but with those men who seize political or anti-political, social or anti-social, economic, or physical power without restraint of their desires. It is this version of man which the majority of us, ourselves engendered, find attractive, and it is the phallic illusion maintained by such men upon which modern male gender roles are based.

Notes

[1]Cat Stevens, "Father and Son," Tea for the Tillerman, A & M Records.

[2]Michael McKeon, "Historicizing Patriarchy: The Emergence of Gender Difference in England, 1660-1760," Eighteenth-Century Studies 28 (1995): 295-322; Thomas Laqueur, Making Sex: Body and Gender from the Greeks to Freud, (Cambridge, MA: Harvard UP, 1990); Michel Foucault, The History of Sexuality, trans. Robert Hurley (New York: Pantheon, 1978); Lawrence Stone, The Family, Sex and Marriage (New York: Harper, 1977); Eve Kosofsky Sedgwick, Between Men (New York: Columbia UP, 1985); Jeffrey Weeks, Sex, Politics and Society: The Regulation of Sexuality Since 1800 (London: Longman, 1981); Nancy Armstrong, Desire and Domestic Fiction (New York: Oxford UP, 1987); and Terry Eagleton, The Rape of Clarissa (Minneapolis: U of Minn P, 1982).

[3]Ruth H. Bloch, "Untangling the Roots of Modern Sex Roles: A Survey of Four Centuries of Change," Signs 4 (1978) 238.

[4]McKeon 316.

[5]See Jane Spencer, The Rise of the Woman Novelist: From Aphra Behn to Jane Austen (Oxford: Blackwell, 1986); Dale Spender, Mothers of the Novel: 100 Good Women Writers before Jane Austen (New York: Pandora, 1986); Catherine Gallagher, Nobody's Story: The Vanishing Acts of Women Writers in the Marketplace 1670-1820 (Berkeley: U of Cal P, 1994).

[6]Alan Bray, Homosexuality in Renaissance England (London: Gay Men's Press, 1982) and Randolph Trumbach "The Birth of the Queen: Sodomy and the Emergence of Gender Equality in Modern Culture, 1660-1750," Hidden From History: Reclaiming the Gay and Lesbian Past, eds. Martin Bauml Duberman et al. (New York: NAL Books, 1989).

[7]Lyndal Roper, Oedipus and the Devil: Witchcraft, Sexuality and Religion in Early Modern Europe (London: Routledge, 1994) 9.

[8]Foucault 26.

[9]Foucault 37.

[10]Roy Porter, "Mixed Feelings: The Enlightenment and Sexuality in Eighteenth-Century Britain," Sexuality in Eighteenth-Century Britain, ed. Paul-Gabriel Boucé (Manchester: Manchester U P, 1982) 1-27, 8.

[11]Porter 21.

[12]Eric Trudgill, Madonnas and Magdalens: The Origins and Development of Victorian Sexual Attitudes (New York: Holmes & Meier, 1976) 160.

[13]Trudgill 160.

[14]Foucault 23.

[15]Armstrong 59.

[16]See particularly Armstrong 14-15, although she argues the novel as an agent of female identification throughout her text.

[17]Laqueur 22.

[18]Laqueur 23.

[19]Foucault 104.

[20]Foucault 37.

[21]Laqueur 11.

[22]See Laqueur and McKeon.

[23]McKeon 295.

[24]See Kate Millett, Sexual Politics (Garden City, NY: Doubleday, 1970) for a historical background covering the beginnings of feminism and what Millett terms the sexual revolution.

[25]Laqueur 22.

[26]Armstrong refers to the "power of surveillance" which she also terms "panoptical power," 22. This power, she argues, displaces the aristocratic power of the body to hold the gaze and was, therefore, superior to the gaze during this earlier time, 123.

[27]Straub, Sexual Suspects: Eighteenth-Century Players and Sexual Ideology (Princeton: Princeton UP, 1992) 19.

[28]McKeon 314.

[29]McKeon 301.

[30]McKeon 315.

[31]One of the principle advocates of this position is Rousseau, with whose views Mary Wollstonecraft argues in A Vindication of the Rights of Woman, A Mary Wollstonecraft Reader, eds. Barbara H. Solomon and Paula S. Berggren (New York: Mentor, 1983).

[32]McKeon takes these classes of men from one of Richard Steele's papers in The Tatler, 312-313.

[33]Robert Markley, Fallen Languages (Ithaca: Cornell UP, 1993) 27.

[34]McKeon 315.

[35]Christopher Hill, <u>Some Intellectual Consequences of the English Revolution</u> (Madison: U of Wisc P, 1980) 7.

[36]Hill 34.

[37]Hugh Ross Williamson, <u>The Day They Killed the King</u> (London: Frederick Muller, 1957).

[38]Hill 3.

[39]Sigmund Freud, <u>Totem and Taboo and Other Works</u>, vol XIII of <u>The Complete Psychological Works</u> (London: Hogarth, 1955, 1981) 145.

[40]Freud 149.

[41]Freud 151.

[42]Carol Pateman, <u>The Sexual Contract</u> (Stanford: Stanford UP, 1988); see particularly her Chapter Four, "Genesis, Fathers and the Political Liberty of Sons," 77-115, which discusses Freud's primal father, Fulmer's patriarch, and the arguments of Locke and Rousseau against absolutism and for the social (and, therefore, sexual) contract.

[43]Pateman 77.

[44]Pateman 99.

[45]See Sedgwick.

[46]John Locke, <u>Of Civil Government, Second Treatise</u> (Chicago: Gateway, 1955) 4-13.

[47]Locke 109.

[48]Linda J. Nicholson, <u>Gender and History: The Limits of Social Theory in the Age of the Family</u> (New York: Columbia UP, 1986) 133-166.

[49]Nicholson 161.

[50]Edmund Burke, <u>Reflections on the Revolution in France,</u> ed. Thomas H. D. Mahoney (New York: Macmillan, 1955) 68.

[51]Burke 50.

[52]Burke 87.

[53]Burke 102.

[54]Hill 3.

[55]Nicholson 134.

[56]Locke 177.

[57]Locke 77.

[58]For an analysis of Filmer's arguments and Locke's rebuttal, see Nicholson 133 and Pateman 85-96.

[59]Jonathan Scott Lee, Jacques Lacan (Amherst: U of MA P, 1990) 15.

[60]Jacques Lacan, Ecrits, trans. Alan Sheridan (New York: Norton, 1977) 285.

[61]Lacan, from Seminar 20, quoted in Lee 175.

[62]Lacan, 290.

[63]Lawrence Stone, The Past and Present Revisited (1981; London: Routledge, 1987) 222-240.

[64]Stone, 229.

[65]tone, especially 227 and 245.

[66]Randolph Trumbach, "London's Sodomites: Homosexual Behavior and Western Culture in the Eighteenth Century, Journal of Social History 11 (1977) 1-33.

[67]Trumbach, "London's Sodomites," 13.

[68]Kaja Silverman, Male Subjectivity at the Margins (New York: Routledge, 1992) 15.

[69]Susan Dwyer Amussen, An Ordered Society: Gender and Class in Early Modern England (Oxford: Basil Blackwell, 1988) 120.

[70]Mary Wollstonecraft, A Vindication of the Rights of Woman, A Mary Wollstonecraft Reader, eds. Barbara H. Solomon and Paula S. Berggren (New York: Mentor, 1983) 268.

[71]Sedgwick 33.

[72]Fanny Burney, Evelina or, A Young Lady's Entrance into the World (London: Dent, 1958) 235.

[73]Armstrong 4.

[74]Armstrong 14-15.

[75]Eagleton 13.

[76]Armstong 20.

[77]Bray points out how male homosexuality, while always regarded as aberrant and even demonic, was generally not prosecuted as the crime it was considered until the late seventeenth century. At that time, the Societies for the Reformation of Manners began to enforce the law against male homosexuality. Seemingly, to Bray, a haphazard and irregular persecution of "mollies," or male homosexuals began at the same time that these mollies began to form their own urban culture. The change he sees is one of identification. Prior to this time, homosexual acts were something which just happened as part of the lived experience, but once society began to prosecute those who committed homosexual acts, a homosexual identity evolved as a means of defense which both protected and alienated the individual.

[78]McKeon 308-310.

[79]Eagleton 6.

[80]Eagleton 15.

[81]Trudgill briefly discusses this give and take between the growing middle class and the aristocracy by noting how middle-class sexual attitudes influenced the aristocracy which, in turn, provided an example for the middle-class, 160.

[82]Freud defines the perversions in The Three Essays, A Case of Hysteria, Three Essays on Sexuality and Other Works. Vol VII of The Complete Psychological Works, London: Hogarth, 1953, 1981, 150, but see also 151-160.

[83]Foucault 104.

[84]J. A. Sharpe, Early Modern England: A Social History 1550-1760 (London: Edward Arnold, 1987)78.

[85]Sharpe 119.

[86]Sharpe 149.

[87]Sharpe 188.

[88]Sharpe 220.

[89]Sharpe 195.

[90]Samuel Richardson, The History of Sir Charles Grandison, ed. Jocelyn Harris, vol. I (London: Oxford, 1972) 4.

[91]William Godwin, The Enquirer: Reflections on Education, Manners and Literature (New York: August M. Kelley, 1965) 134.

CHAPTER IV

LOVELACE'S RAPE

Our boys are prudent too soon. . . . their pleasures are those of
hackneyed vice, blunted to every finer emotion by the repetition
of debauch . . . .

> Harley, Henry Mackensie's "Man of Feeling"[1]

The novels of Samuel Richardson mark a transition between the
two types of the early eighteenth century's "female novel of love, . . .
the seduction/rape tale and the courtship novel,"[2] and the later
eighteenth century's Gothic and sentimental novels. According to
Margaret Doody, Richardson's changes in the female novel of love
are associated with his maleness; therefore, "[i]n Richardson's
hands, this type of fiction becomes more robust and more masculine,
[and] male characters and male points of view balance the central
female interest."[3] Later, in the hands of male Gothic writers such as
Horace Walpole, Matthew Lewis, and William Godwin, this masculine
perspective takes a less balanced approach, and their Gothic novels
center on a ruthless and powerful male villain (or, in Godwin's case, a
villainous system of male relationships) rather than on his female
victim.[4] Nevertheless, Richardson's notorious rake, Robert Lovelace,
seemingly serves as a model for these later male characters,[5] and
Lovelace's example of a predatory and phallic masculinity reappears
in the form of a Manfred, an Ambrosio, and, to a lesser degree, a
Tyrrel or Falkland. In spite of the awful results of Lovelace's behavior, his type of masculinity attracted and interested readers, and

male Gothic writers, by increasing the attention placed upon the villain, made use of this interest. In short, the earlier seduction/rape tale utilized the attraction of the helpless woman to the libertine, or what Doody calls "this fascination of the rabbit by the snake."[6] Richardson developed this attraction when he presented the inner thoughts and, consequently, the motivations of both the rabbit and the snake; subsequently, drawing upon Richardson's example, male Gothic writers used the fascination of the snake to captivate not only the rabbit but the reader as well.

Eighteenth century readers had reasons to recognize a male-dominated world outside the home as a place of growing hostility and danger where circumstances favored resourceful and persever-ant men such as Lovelace and the Gothic villains. Industrialization, urbanization, and the violence of the French Revolution had changed and was changing the face of society, and Gothic fiction is not just about haunted castles, but about this "haunted society."[7] Many could view the world as more dangerous, but even if the world were not more dangerous, the increased availability of reports of disastrous events made it appear so. As Wordsworth suggests in his <u>Preface</u> to the <u>Lyrical Ballads</u> of 1800, improved communication of the events which surrounded these social changes was numbing the minds of individuals to tales of terrible misfortune,[8] and public taste as well as human relationships appeared to be changing to correspond with this increased sense of impending catastrophe and continued competition. Men and women who had relied upon each other in the interdependent commercial world of the village began to see the 'other' as an undependable outsider and a competitor for individual gain rather than as a mutual contributor to the community. In the words of Elizabeth Kraft, "the forces of commercialization had begun to render the changes in society that eventuate in the loss of true sociability, of pleasure in the company of strangers."[9] Social relation-ships which had previously been decided by a person's status at birth were increasingly determined by the wealth that an individual could accumulate or retain. But this possibility of social movement had its own horrors because while a free market economy allowed for men to rise in class and attain a social standing previously unknown to their families, this same precarious marketplace also created the opportunity for men to lose everything. At the same time that more men could consider themselves as upwardly mobile, they were burdened with that potential for improvement and with the possibility that someone else could take everything away. As Godwin demonstrates in Caleb Williams,[10] the greatest modern horror was the social dynamic which pitted man against man, and the man most equipped to win this battle was intelligent and clever, unrelenting and merciless, as well as possessed of an authoritative or striking physical presence. Richardson's Lovelace, a model for the Gothic villains, epitomizes this type of masculinity.

This connection between an emerging masculine type and the changing social conditions is especially important because at the same time that Richardson incorporates a more masculine view-point, he also advances middle-class ideology, a point which Terry Eagleton discusses at length in The Rape of Clarissa. Furthermore, even this economic and social emphasis has its sexual implications, and Eagleton sees Richardson's novels as moving toward (in Sir Charles Grandison) "the production of a new kind of male subject," because "Richardson has grasped the point that the so-called 'woman question' is nothing of the kind--that the root of the sexual problem is men."[11] Nevertheless, while Richardson plays a leading part in the promotion of "middle-class sexual attitudes,"[12] he fails, according to Eagleton, to produce an exemplary male because of the "genuine ideological dilemma" caused by Grandison's virtuously demonstrated male power. While Grandison possesses what are traditionally regarded as feminine virtues (with the values of thrift, peace, and chastity), "he can exercise such virtues precisely because he has power--because he is a paternalist patriarch with a steady flow of cash, deserving poor and faulty friends to be regularly overwhelmed by his forgiveness."[13] Thus, Sir Charles Grandison, Richardson's "Man of Religion and Virtue,"[14] represents an attempt to present an example of virtuous masculinity, but this attempt is inherently flawed because Richardson must provide Sir Charles with some type of male power in order for the character to be recognized as masculine. By creating a Grandison, Richardson hoped to present a morally superior male character who could equal the heroines of his first two novels, Pamela and Clarissa, but Richardson could not escape associating the male with an empowering phallic authority. In effect, the only difference between Lovelace and Grandison is that Sir Charles is unquestionably assumed to have the same power which Lovelace works so hard to prove he possesses. In terms of dynamics, however, Lovelace, in his efforts to possess what he desires, provides a clearer and more interesting example of an active masculinity than Sir Charles, who begins the novel "already perfect" and "is bound to be static."[15]

In order to understand the attraction of Lovelace, however, it is necessary to examine how the invention of a Sir Charles underscores Richardson's concern with his earlier male creation. As Tom Keymer notes, "Richardson was acutely aware of the problem"[16] he had created in Lovelace. In trying to undo the power of his earlier creation, Richardson pays homage to the endurance of the evil character by recreating him in a virtuous man. Lovelace provides the model for so many of Sir Charles's strengths that, in Frankenstein-like fashion, the monster emerges as a force against which his creator operates. The second creation, Sir Charles, seems a determined effort to reconcile the influence of the first. In order to be superior to Lovelace, the character of Sir Charles must begin with all the positive characteristics of his predecessor. "Sir Charles was made both handsome and well-dressed against all Richardson's convictions that virtue did not need an outward beauty"[17] because producing a hero with physical qualities which were less than perfection ran the risk of a negative comparison to Lovelace. Lovelace sets the standard for masculinity that his successor must equal. The true test of manhood for Sir Charles comes in a comparison not with Sir Hargrave and the other lesser males of the later novel, but with Lovelace, the earlier character and his prototype. In much the same way that Sir Charles must, in the story, live down the profligacy of his father, Sir Thomas, the character of Sir Charles must overcome the reputation of his notorious fictional ancestor.[18]

Though Sir Charles "controls and directs the world with the authority of virtue, in contrast to Lovelace's control of his world through perverted ingenuity,"[19] Richardson presents both male characters in control. In terms of the male hierarchy, the virtuous Sir Charles and the evil Lovelace occupy the same position as representatives of a controlling manhood in spite of their contrasting behavior. Sir Charles shares Lovelace's "verbal skills and ability to control people"[20] and is admired, like Lovelace, by both men and women. In addition, while Sir Charles's conduct is virtuous because he selflessly protects Harriet by keeping her domiciled,[21] and Lovelace's behavior is immoral because he imprisons Clarissa for his own selfish purposes, both men secure a woman inside while they wander free outside. Lovelace's frequently feigned protection of Clarissa from her father, her brother, her uncles, or their operatives demonstrates, however, how closely male protection resembles imprisonment. In a sense, one measure of Sir Charles's manhood (like Lovelace's) is his ability (or inability) to keep his woman safely at home. Consequently, Sir Charles's virtue is rewarded when Harriet marries him and stays in his home whereas Lovelace loses everything, including his life, after Clarissa escapes him.

In the world outside the home, Sir Charles also shares Lovelace's ability to violently overcome other men, a quality Richardson presents during the first appearance of Sir Charles through Sir Charles's description of his rescue of Harriet from Sir Hargrave Pollexfen:

> Sir Hargrave drew his sword, which he had held between his knees in the scabbard . . . .
>
> "I opened the chariot-door. Sir Hargrave made a pass at me. Take that, and be damn'd to you, for your insolence, scoundrel! said he.
>
> "I was aware of his thrust, and put it by; but his sword a little raked my shoulder.
>
> "My sword was in my hand; but undrawn.
>
> "The chariot-door remaining open (I was not so ceremonious, as to let down the foot-step to take the gentleman out) I seized him by the collar before he could recover himself from the pass he had made at me; and with a jerk, and a kind of twist, laid him under the hind-wheel of his chariot.
>
> "I wrench'd his sword from him, and snapp'd it, and flung the two pieces over my head."[22]

In this passage Sir Charles demonstrates his superior masculinity through his easy dismissal of Sir Hargrave's violent attack. Sir Charles, who has a sword but does not have to use it, merely avoids the thrust of Sir Hargrave's phallic blade, a weapon drawn from between his knees. Instead of retaliating in a similarly malicious fashion, Sir Charles breaks his adversary's sword, an act which after

110

the conflict leaves him not only the better swordsman, but the only swordsman. Sir Charles does not just defeat his opponent; he lays him on the ground and symbolically castrates him.[23] While Sir Charles displays his virtue by demonstrating his restraint and lack of desire for conflict, he is able to do so only because he is unquestionably the better man. Doody is correct when she states that "the frightening thing about him is that he is too independent, too invulnerable."[24] Unlike Sir Hargrave and Lovelace, Sir Charles does not need to work to dominate others; he begins the novel as the superior male. As a man, Sir Charles already has a completeness and an unassailability that others lack; he is too much like God.

In creating such a hypermasculine character as Sir Charles, Richardson attempted to redirect the attraction which readers had for Lovelace toward the character of a good man, but whether or not Richardson succeeded remains debatable. Although Grandison may have been more immediately popular than Clarissa,[25] Richardson's final novel "is generally considered the stepbrother of [his] other novels, a disappointment after the triumph of Clarissa."[26] While the critical assessment and overall popularity of these novels depend on several factors, the tension created by Lovelace's evil presence in Clarissa maintains a level of excitement that the later novel lacks. Furthermore, the balanced male/female perspective in the earlier novel is lost in Grandison because Sir Charles's humility will not allow him repeatedly to sing his own praises, and "the emphasis is thrown on the female characters,"[27] especially Harriet, who tells the bulk of the story.

In Clarissa, until the rape scene in what was originally volume five, Lovelace manipulates the other characters, and his power captivates both Clarissa and the reader. Sales declined for those volumes subsequent to and including the rape,[28] and this trend in sales can lead to Keymer's conclusion that "Richardson's novels prospered or declined in proportion with their heroines;"[29] however, this reduced interest may also be related to the decline of Lovelace, whose masculine identity suffers after Clarissa escapes him. Nevertheless, Lovelace's model of evil masculinity was so compelling to readers that even during the process of writing Clarissa, Richardson attempted to rewrite the character to diminish his appeal. The serial publication of Clarissa, "at three different periods of time" (IV 552),[30] had provided Richardson with an opportunity to receive reader responses during the process of writing the novel, and women readers, in particular, begged him to write a happy ending by "reforming Lovelace, and marrying him to Clarissa" (IV 552). In his letters, he "complains repeatedly of women's favorable responses to the villainous Lovelace,"[31] and he wrote a postscript to the novel in order to explain his reasons for retaining the tragic conclusion. His purpose in the novel, he writes, had been to "investigate the great doctrines of Christianity," and

> he could not bear . . . to have a Lovelace for a series of years glory in his wickedness, and think that he had nothing to do, but as an act of grace and favour to hold out his hand to receive that of the best of women, whenever he pleased, and to have it thought, that marriage would be a sufficient amends for all his enormities to others, as well as to her. (IV 553)

Still, Richardson found himself defending Clarissa, whom some readers thought "too cold in her love, too haughty, and even sometimes provoking" (IV 558), and vilifying Lovelace in an effort to prove his point. During the writing of the novel, he modified Lovelace's behavior to make him more evil. In a letter to Lady Bradshaigh, he admits:

> I thought I had made him too wicked, too intriguing, too revengeful, (and that in his very first letters) for him to obtain the favour and good wishes of any worthy heart of either sex. I try'd his

character, as it was first drawn, and his last exit, on a young lady of seventeen. She shewed me by her tears at the latter that he was not very odious to her for vagaries and inventions. I was surprized; and for fear such a wretch should induce pity, I threw into his character some deeper shades.[32]

Lovelace, however, remained a fascinating character, so Richardson keeps reminding his readers of the horrible death the libertine suffers. In the "Postscript" to Clarissa, he describes painting "the death of the wicked, as terrible as he could paint it" (IV 554), and, in the "Preface" to Grandison, he reminds his readers of the "wretched and disappointed"[33] Lovelace who "perishes miserably in the bloom of life, and sinks into the grave oppressed with guilt, remorse, and horror."[34] Nevertheless, Lovelace's horrible death does not necessarily erase the appeal of his life. By creating a male character charismatic and devious enough to interest and manipulate Clarissa, Richardson also presents a version of masculinity which attracts readers. Though readers may inevitably agree with Richardson's moral conclusions about Lovelace's character, the possibility of this attraction remains. In spite of the author's intentions, Lovelace's masculinity appears to be the primary masculinity promoted by the novel.

Richardson needed a strong, male figure to test his heroine, but, as Keymer points out in his comparison of various contemporary reactions, Richardson tests his audience as well. "The novel's readers remain free to 'carve' a variety of routes" which include an "embrace [of] all that Lovelace offers."[35] Why, however, do many readers ignore all of "Richardson's envisaged paths toward repudiation"[36] of Lovelace? The simple answer is that structurally Richardson places Lovelace in a position of unchallenged phallic power and develops his character by showing multiple manifestations of that power. Like Sir Charles, Lovelace has formed his masculine reputation before the events of the novel, but unlike Sir Charles, whose reputation allows him to maintain his role as the superior male without dueling or taking advantage of the women who love him, Lovelace actively asserts his authority and revels in his accomplishments. At the beginning of Clarissa, Lovelace has already proved the significance of his masculinity in comparison to other men and in his relationships with women, and the early action of the novel confirms his superiority. He initially outduels James Harlowe, Jr. and his continued threat to challenge James Jr. and other males in the Harlowe circle is used to induce Clarissa to continue her correspondence with him (I 85). Lovelace is also "leader" (I 151) of the rakes, a position which establishes him as superior to both the men he associates with and the women he has "taught to dress, and helped to undress" (I 511). His question to Belford, "am I not likely to be thy king and thy emperor in the great affair before us?" (I 152), is rhetorical. Lovelace recognizes himself as the king, the premier male, among his acquaintance, and his character holds that ultimate rank in the novel. The focus of Clarissa may be the heroine's selfhood,[37] but the plot unfolds amid competing masculinities and Lovelace occupies the strongest masculine position of all.

In order to develop an atmosphere of enclosure and danger for his heroine, Richardson placed her in the midst of conflicting male powers. For the first quarter of the text, from the beginning until the moment Clarissa flees with Lovelace, readers share Clarissa's difficult choice between parental authority and her desire for something other than what her parents offer. Until Lovelace tricks Clarissa into leaving with him, parental authority represented by Clarissa's father, brother, uncles, and "masculine" (I 386) sister prohibits and keeps her from pursuing the unknown, outside enjoyments represented by Lovelace, the "man of pleasure" (I 49). Clarissa eventually rejects both of these worldly choices and neither pursues the possible pleasures which

Lovelace promises nor accepts the mandates from her parents, but, by choosing a life beyond the grave, she also abandons any earthly desires she may have possessed. Clarissa's physical alternatives require her to surrender herself to one male authority or another because both the inner circle of the Harlowes and the outer domain of Lovelace are controlled by men, and she is only able to escape this control by spiritually rising above this male dominion.

Caught between the odious demands of her family and the immoral overtures of Lovelace, Clarissa is unable to reach a compromise in marriage. She must instead deal with the conflicting desires of the male world which surrounds her while, at the same time, wanting or desiring something else. Initially, Lovelace has the potential to fulfill her desires, and until she flees with him, he represents both the mysterious object of desire and her probable ruin. By constructing an outer, unknown world of promise and threat around an inner circle of restraint and the denial of pleasure, Richardson places both Clarissa and the reader in this position between desire and authority. In Lacanian terms, this location between unknown, forbidden pleasures (a) and the ideal world where master signifiers provide completeness (S1) which is organized into a system of signifiers (S2) corresponds to the position of those experiencing hysterical neurosis.[38] As the subject unwilling to accept the doctrine of the master, yet unable to produce her own signifier for her own desire, Clarissa (and with her the reader) remains divided ($) between the master signifier (obedience) which is offered to complete her and that which she believes she lacks. For approximately the first quarter of the novel, Richardson maintains the tension of this discourse, the Discourse of the Hysteric:[39]

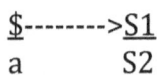

$$\frac{\$}{a} \text{-------->} \frac{S1}{S2}$$

115

In this initial section of the text, Richardson provides neither Clarissa nor the reader with an option that will resolve this fundamental split ($) between Clarissa's desire (a) to choose for herself and the demand that she obey the word of the master (S1). The master signifier "parental authority" which is allied to the "prerogative of manhood" (I 61) is the symbolic point on which Clarissa's (and the reader's) alienation pivots. The rupture in her familial relations occurs because she refuses to obey the word of her father (I 37), and by refusing obedience indicates a desire for something else. While Clarissa repeatedly states that this desire is to be able to signify her own desire (and thus end her alienation) through assertion of her right to control the fate of her body, her family insists that her desire is for Lovelace. In effect, the Harlowes deny the possibility of female desire and privilege the phallus, embodied by Lovelace, as the signifier of male desire, the only desire which they can recognize. Like Clarissa, readers are not provided a choice other than parental authority and phallic power, and when the master signifiers of parental authority are questioned, readers, too, experience the uncomfortable feeling of not knowing which values to accept.

In opposition to the word of Clarissa's father stands the figure of Lovelace. Possessing a masculinity which allows him seemingly easy access to all but Clarissa, the best of women, Lovelace represents phallic power. He stands at the top of the male hierarchy, and only his own dissatisfaction with himself can bring about his death. As the manipulative "director" of the "principal motions" (I 494) of the Harlowes, Lovelace controls Clarissa's body from the outset, and he also controls the outside or male world of the novel, a world of violence and pretense. Lovelace's duel with Clarissa's brother James described in the first letter initiates all the subsequent events, and his death occurs in the final letter, twenty-six letters after Clarissa's death has been described by Belford. In addition to constantly scheming ways in which to exercise his will with Clarissa, Lovelace also lies to her, forges letters, and often disguises himself. In contrast to the Harlowes, who rely on the power of their static word to enlist Clarissa's obedience, Lovelace demonstrates an ambiguity which makes him initially difficult for Clarissa to define. All that is known is that he has a power and seemingly possesses something that others lack.

When the Harlowes expressly forbid Clarissa to have contact with Lovelace, they identify him with that which is excluded by their language and law. Consequently, Lovelace occupies the position of the object <u>a</u> as a source of *jouissance* forbidden by the master signifiers of the Symbolic Order authority of Clarissa's parents and represents the object (<u>a</u>) of fantasy for the readers and Clarissa. The divided subject's ($) desire for an unknown *jouissance* or "*the plus-de -jouir* (<u>a</u>), a surplus of *jouissance* over and above what the subject currently attains,"[40] results in fantasy ($ <> <u>a</u>), the subject's relationship with its want-of-being. In this case, Clarissa's (and the reader's) desire for a way around her parent's mandates seems answered by the promise of Lovelace, who not only offers an alternative to the parental discourse but also represents a forbidden pleasure. He seemingly holds the secret to the phallus, the signifier for desire which is left out of the Symbolic and Imaginary Registers. The more oppressively Clarissa's family restricts her correspondence (her Symbolic expression) and her movement (her Imaginary freedom), the more attractive Lovelace becomes.

When Clarissa begins to consider Lovelace as an alternative, she is seeking a way out of these Symbolic and Imaginary restraints. Comparing a life with Lovelace to that with her family, she asks Anna, "At worst, will he confine me prisoner to my chamber? Will he deny me the visits of my dearest friend, and forbid me to correspond with her?" (I 200) Ironically, Lovelace will eventually hold her captive and interfere with her correspondence, but what is important to Clarissa in this passage is not the actual Lovelace but the symbol of completion and security which he represents. He is, she admits, "brave" and "generous," and she is tempted by her family, her "cruel friends," to "try the difference" (I 200). Furthermore, he promises to help her escape to the independence of a private lodging (I 452) and, by doing so, offers the possibility of fulfilling what she perceives as her lack in ways which can be described in all three Lacanian registers, the Symbolic, the Imaginary, and the Real.

At the Symbolic level, she identifies the signifiers of "reconciliation," "liberty," and "free will" (I 442) as those which she desires in place of the "obedience" her parents demand. At the Imaginary level, she seeks to free her physical image from confinement and to avoid the image of the "horrid wretch" (I 42) Mr. Solmes, whose "ugly weight" had "so offended" her that she had "involuntarily" lost "command" over herself (I 68). In place of this Imaginary position, Lovelace offers her the image of physical freedom and the presence of what Clarissa describes as "the gracefulness of his figure" (I 446). At the same time, on the level of the Real, Lovelace's character suggests a *jouissance* alien and undefinable to Clarissa's Symbolic and Imaginary experience. In addition to being at the top of the male hierarchy, having a fine figure, and possessing a good fortune (I 199), he is Clarissa's "secret" (I 45), the embodiment of what she cannot express in language. Anna, too, is unable to describe him adequately. "What can you do," she asks, "with or without such an enterprising--?" The blank is left for Clarissa to fill in with "a word bad enough," but she is able only to call him "the vilest of men" (I 352), a phrase which operates like "the king of the rakes" to further assert Lovelace's masculine superiority and phallic position.

In actuality, these expressions serve only to support Lovelace's superlative position, and Clarissa's continued inability to define him or to decide what to do "with or without" him sustains the audience's belief that he is what she lacks. Their union appears inevitable. After Clarissa flees with Lovelace, Anna's repeated advice to "delay not the [marriage] ceremony" implies that only one conclusion, Clarissa's seduction, can be drawn from a woman's presence in the company of a man like Lovelace, the representative of masculine power.

Unlike Clarissa, readers are privy to Lovelace's consistently selfish motives and manipulative actions, but they also have no other choice than to hope that he may somehow unite with Clarissa. The alternative put forth by her family (the Symbolic order) and embodied in the image of the hideous Mr. Solmes (the Imaginary register), is not an actual possibility. Clarissa refuses him repeatedly, and her statement, "I never will have that man" (I 436), exemplifies her resolve and confirms the reader's expectations. With the failure of the Symbolic order to provide signifiers which promise security and wholeness, the reader as the divided subject ($) in the position of the hysteric seeks a new master, or set of master signifiers. When Clarissa flees her parents, she and the reader leave the master signifiers connected to parental authority behind. At this point, the reader is left free to examine the value system (S2) proposed by Lovelace as well as the opposing system utilized by Clarissa and adopted by Belford.

Richardson's novel, therefore, begins by utilizing the discourse of the hysteric to create a fundamental split ($) in Clarissa and the reader between the command of the master (S1) and the object of desire (a). After Clarissa resolves this conflict by escaping her parents' confinement, however, she eventually defines her master (S1) as God and her value system (S2) as that established by Christian discourse. In effect, the reader is interpellated through this discourse to the position of the receiver of knowledge in what Lacan calls the Discourse of the University:[41]

$$\frac{S2}{S1} \text{-----> } \frac{a}{\$}$$

The reader, made uncomfortable or anxious by the Discourse of the Hysteric and with an identification with the alienated Clarissa ($\$$), seeks to resolve this anxiety by adopting a discourse which furnishes a master signifier or signifiers which, in turn, answer the riddle of desire ($\underline{a}$) by supplying a system of knowledge (S2). Richardson's solution is to offer Christian discourse (S2) as the answer, and readers may accept this alternative; however, the Discourse of the University does not relieve and may even increase the reader's feelings of fundamental alienation ($\$$), and readers may seek the answer to their desire elsewhere in the text in the opposing discourse of Lovelace, whose own value system (S2) also promises a type of fulfillment. While Richardson in the writing and rewriting of Clarissa promotes the former discourse through his heroine, he continues to offer the villain's discourse as a wicked alternative. The maintenance of the two discourses allows the reader ample time to measure both sides. As Doody points out, "[the] personal imperial principle manifested in Lovelace's will, and Clarissa's Christain morality are curiously parallel."[42] Though Richardson may expect the reader to recognize that "the Christian spirit, by the power of God's love, is always free, and this true freedom transcends the life of power and conquest,"[43] there is nothing to prevent the reader from considering Lovelace's propositions and arguments. Indeed, the position of phallic power from which Lovelace operates makes his alternative discourse attractive to those inclined to value physical rewards over spiritual ones. He seems to be able to possess all that he desires.

For the remainder of the text, these two different sets of master signifiers, those of Lovelace and those of Clarissa, Belford, Anna Howe, and the other characters who become allied against Lovelace, promote conflicting value systems. Lovelace wages an "amorous warfare" (I 514) for his "predominant passion" of "girl not gold" (II 20) while the competing discourse urges "marriage" until the rape, then emphasizes "death." In turn, Lovelace is defined not only by his desire for Clarissa but by his opposition to her discourse. Opposition, in fact, is an important signifier in Lovelace's discourse. "I love opposition" (II 185), he states, and when he taunts Hickman with the identity of Clarissa's other lover "DEATH" (III 495), he acknowledges his adversarial relationship to both the discourse of death and to death itself. Correspondingly, he will fight his final battle with Colonel Morden (derived from the Latin "mors" or "mort") whose name "announces his symbolic meaning" as the "representation of Death."[44] In the meantime, he does everything possible to maintain his discourse of a conquering, independent male desire, denying not only death but marriage as well. His question, "What shall we say if all were to mean nothing but MATRIMONY?" (II 32) signifies his own ontological position. Marriage, to Lovelace, means the abandonment of male desire and, subsequently, the recognition of castration and death. By substituting the signifiers of male conquest and control in the place of an unsatisfiable desire, he is able to hide his want-of-being (his castration and mortality) from himself in the rules (I 171) and language of the rake. He predicates his existence on a belief in sexual conquest and the male camaraderie embodied in his wit and friendship with his fellow rakes. The signifiers (S1) for the female, or other, sex like "girl" or "that sex" take the place for Lovelace of the object of desire (the object a), and the system of knowledge (S2) which he promulgates with these signifiers allows him to hide from his own castration or want-of-being.

In effect, Lovelace's master discourse uses the master signifiers (S1) of male subjugation and domination to form a code (S2) of conduct which covers over his actual desires (a) and denies his alienation ($) in what Lacan calls the Discourse of the Master.[45]

$$\underline{S1} \text{-----}> \underline{S2}$$
$$\$ \qquad a$$

In Lovelace's discourse, males are active assayers and females are passive respondents: "Men are to ask; women are to deny" (II 185). Lovelace's preference for the "pursuit and conquest of a fine woman to all the joys of life" (I 249) not only reasserts the active nature of his masculinity and his view of the passive, objectified position of women, but also indicates the importance of the signifier, "fine woman," to the maintenance of this masculinity. Defining "fine woman," however, creates a dilemma. For example, Lovelace realizes too late that Clarissa is the ultimate "fine woman" because of her steadfast refusal of his advances, even when she is drugged almost senseless and raped. Nevertheless, if she is not tested past the point of physical penetration, Lovelace would not know her limits. The rape reveals the flaw in Lovelace's system and the fantasy ($ <> a) that is subordinated by his master discourse. The "fine woman" he is seeking is the realization of desire, possession of the object $\underline{a}$, itself and, by definition, unobtainable. Lovelace's belief that possession of Clarissa's body will mean something denies the impossibility of this fantasy. Only when Clarissa herself, and not her body, proves to be unobtainable, does Lovelace recognize that she is what he wants and also that she represents an even greater significance, "the cause of God" (IV 91). His libertine discourse is undone by the recognition that he has missed not just a possible marriage with this best of women, but the immortality offered by a union with God. Faced with the breakdown of his own belief system, Lovelace begins to understand and accept the discourse of his opponents.

On this level of signifiers, readers also generally accept the moral conclusion. Lovelace, as Richardson points out, does not deserve Clarissa. Any man who utilizes woman after woman as the object of a sport which reinforces a narcissistic male identity has not earned the right to be linked with the best of women. Yet, on the deeper level of desire, Lovelace's motives are ambiguous and the reader's reactions more complicated. While Lovelace continuously besieges the body of Clarissa, he is seeking more than physical conquest. As his name indicates, he also wants love, and Clarissa refuses "to acknowledge that love" (II 38). Beneath this game of pursuit and conquest of the fine woman lies the desire to be loved for oneself, and this desire extends beyond the love of individual men and women to the love of the Symbolic Other, "the ultimate authority or source of meaning."[46] In other words, Lovelace pursues the love of women through offering what he views as a "mask" (II 471) in the form of his manipulative inventions, wit, wealth, social status, and physical appeal; consequently, he finds the hidden part of himself, that part which is not a fictional invention, never loved. Clarissa's rejection of his constructed identity implies that she understands the identity beneath this mask. Her acknowledgments to Anna Howe that "I have owned more than once . . . that I could have liked Mr. Lovelace above all men" (II 438) and to Belford that "I once could have loved him" (IV 306) hint that something exists beneath Lovelace's facade that Clarissa could love. Clarissa, however, changes from "woman to angel"[47] only by denying not just Lovelace, but the entire male world of the novel. When Clarissa ascends to the status of Symbolic Other, however, Lovelace can only recognize his failure to attain what he really wanted: the sanctioning love (and, by extension, immortality) granted by the Symbolic Other.

Throughout the entire novel, therefore, Lovelace remains on the outside. Unable to accept the values of the "old patriarchal system," which tells him that sex should by limited to the "matrimonial state" for the purposes of "contributing to get sons and daughters" (III 316), Lovelace resists Lord M's declaration that "you will marry, as your father, and all your ancestors, did before you: else you would have had no title to be my heir; nor can your descendants have any title to be yours, unless they are legitimate" (II 408). By rejecting the patriarchal system, Lovelace represents a new type of masculinity. Instead of yielding to Lord M's will and relying on the title of his ancestors to supply him with a male authority, Lovelace creates himself and controls the world around him through his belief in the sufficiency of heterosexual male desire and his opposition to the discourse of sexual denial, marriage, and death. Though the system he creates fails in the novel, he remains a attractive character for readers because he suggests a possible alternative to castration and death. Outside of the Symbolic order and the authority of the father, he has access to unlimited sexual pleasure. He and his fellow rakes have "pursued from pretty girl to pretty girl, as fast as we had set one down, taking another up" (III 316), and, until he meets Clarissa, he has no reason to discontinue this practice. Clarissa castrates Lovelace, as he, like Oedipus, becomes sightless: "Clarissa has made me eyeless and senseless to every other beauty" (III 392); however, his recognition of his lack does not eliminate the possibility that he might have become whole through a union with Clarissa. "Wanting her, I want my own soul" (II 524), he says when she escapes at the end of the original volume IV, and the reader understands that what Lovelace desires is a state beyond sexual union or marital union or any condition offered by the Symbolic order. He wants to be complete and uncastrated in the world outside of images and language.

Furthermore, as the only male who could be loved by Clarissa, Lovelace remains potentially able to achieve that state.

In opposition to Lovelace, the moral discourse of the novel promotes a system of knowledge (S2) that uses the master signifiers (S1) of "marriage" and "death" to conceal desire ($\underline{a}$) and to encourage the reader away from recognition of his/her castrated condition ($) and toward acceptance of this system of knowledge. In this Master Discourse

$$\underline{S1} \text{ -----> } \underline{S2}$$
$$\$ \qquad a$$

the signifiers of "death" and "marriage" are defined and differentiated at the level of the Imaginary. Good conduct is rewarded by an absence of physical pain, and the "good" characters receive happy marriages or blissful deaths. Anna Howe "esteem[s] and love[s]" (IV 548) Hickman and he is "affectionate" to her, and "they are already blessed with two fine children" (IV 547). Mrs. Norton does not die, but departs with "ease and calmness" while "falling into a sweet slumber" (IV 547). Belford is made "as completely happy as a man can be" (IV 550) by his marriage to Miss Charlotte Montague. He is also "blessed with a son by her" (IV 550) which, in turn, allows Lord M. to be "pleased" when "at his death" (IV 550) he can bequeath the bulk of his estate to that son. Clarissa experiences the most beautiful death of all, expiring with "a smile" and "such a charming serenity overspreading her sweet face at the instant, as seemed to manifest her eternal happiness already begun" (IV 347).

Contrasted to all these happy deaths and marriages are the images of the dying and poorly married villains. Mrs. Sinclair's "dreadful exit" (IV 536) epitomizes their fate as she dies "more like a wolf than a human creature" (IV 380). The physical images of "her huge quaggy carcass," "her mill-post arms," "her big eyes, goggling and flaming red," her matted grizzly hair . . . spread about her fat ears and brawny neck," "her livid lips parched," "her wide mouth . . . splitting her face, as it were, into two parts," "her huge tongue hideously rolling in it," and "her bellows-shaped and various-coloured breasts" (IV 382) reinforce the painful bodily experience of Sinclair's death and also suggest the hideousness of her sexual nature. The repulsive images of grizzly hair, parched lips, a wide, almost chasmic mouth, and multi-colored breasts contrast with her use of the female body to attract and encourage desire. In this description, the female is a shapeless mass with an orifice which resembles an ominous pit. Mrs. Sinclair is not only a "damned soul already in hell,"[48] she herself is the image of hell at her death. Belton, while he receives more sympathy than Mrs. Sinclair from Belford, also dies in a protracted, horrific manner. In a similar, but much more abbreviated fashion, Sally Martin dies of a fever, Polly Horton dies of a violent cold, and Betty Barnes and Joseph Leman die of consumption. While all of these characters die unmar-ried, James and Arabella live to be married, "but not to take joy in either of their nuptials" (IV 535). Finally, of course, Clarissa's primary antagonist, Lovelace, dies after having "suffered much" and acting "as if he had seen some frightful spectre" (IV 530).

This discourse is designed to interpellate readers into a position where once recognizing that "dying" is "the common lot," they embrace the "Christian" (IV 346) conduct of Clarissa. As Doody has pointed out, Richardson was drawing on a history of devotional literature when he shows, in the novel, how death means something different to the good and the bad characters.[49] For the bad, death is an ominous specter while the good experience death as a welcomed friend. For the reader, however, death is a reminder of non-existence and the fundamental split ($) which occurs through the understand-ing of our mortality. The effectiveness of the moral discourse de-

126

pends upon the reader's acceptance of the Christian code as an escape from non-being. If a reader doubts this code, the discourse may have a limited influence on him or her. In other words, the dramatically contrasted deaths of Clarissa and Mrs. Sinclair have less or little impact on the reader who sees both characters as similarly dead (non-existent). The power of this moral discourse is further weakened by an ambiguous treatment of male characters in the application of the code. Clarissa's conduct provides a clear example of what females should do, and the deaths of the incorrigible female characters demonstrate the disastrous results of a misstep; however, males like Colonel Morden, who duels, and Belford, who has a reputation for sexual misconduct, are not precluded forgiveness and an ultimate reward. While the novel establishes chastity as a metaphor for female virtue, a standard for virtuous male sexuality never gets clearly defined.

Although one of Richardson's stated purposes in the novel is to warn against the "too commonly received notion that a reformed rake makes the best husband,"[50] Belford, Lovelace's lieutenant rake, gets rewarded for his reformation with a wife, a son, and an increased estate by the novel's end. While all of the "sisters in iniquity" (IV 536) die, Belford reforms and prospers, and his fellow rakes Mowbray and Tourville retire to the country. Clarissa reaches the sexual limits of female virtue by being the semi-conscious victim of a rape, and, even then, she makes Lovelace suffer "by her nails and her teeth" (III 200); correspondingly, however, Lovelace appears beyond redemption only because he is worse than every other male. Women seemingly must deny sexual desire and either desire a domestic tranquility (Anna) or a spiritual serenity (Clarissa); on the other hand, men apparently must only bring sexual desire under control by eventually restricting it to one woman.

This presentation of the sexual double standard undermines the moral message of the text. While attacking the phallic discourse of Lovelace, the moral discourse continues to privilege the phallus. The question is not whether male power should exist, but where it originates. For Lovelace, his repeated maxim that a woman "once overcome" is "forever overcome" (III 318) is an example of how he identifies the penis as the subjugator of women and the source of phallic power, but, for Clarissa, "male power . . . rests on social and theological foundations."[51] The forces in conflict, therefore, are not just an evil man versus a set of righteous principles, but an individual, self-created masculinity against a masculinity provided by a higher patriarchal power. Lovelace's fatal error is not his treatment of women or of other men, but his inability to identify a higher power than himself. In contrast, Belford reforms when he realizes his mortality in the deaths of others. Lovelace states to Belford that "thy uncle's slow death, and thy attendance upon him through every stage towards it, prepared thee for [reformation]" (III 496), but Lovelace denies his own death even until his final letter when he "doubt[s] not to be able to write again" (IV 528). In the end, however, Lovelace meets death in his symbolic duel with Colonel Morden, another masculine figure. This meeting has already been foreshadowed by Lovelace's dream (IV 136) where Morden appears with his sword drawn and is abetted by Lord M who throws his "great black mantle" over Lovelace's head. While the moral is provided in the dream by Lovelace's fall into the hole of Elden, the confrontation remains between Lovelace and a representative of the patriarchal hierarchy that he resists. In the novel, life and death as well as salvation and perdition are decided by one's subservience to this higher male authority.

While Richardson clearly wants his audience to accept the promise of immortality in "the region of seraphims" with its "golden cherubs and glittering seraphs" (IV 136), readers remain free to weigh their own interests in this battle of competing masculinities and masculine discourses. Even if readers identify with the moral message at the level of the Symbolic and wish, in the Imaginary register, to choose a peaceful death over the horrific bodily endings of the villains, they may identify with the fantasy of phallic totality symbolized by Lovelace in the earthly world which competes with the fantasy of immortality in the clouds. The moral discourse instructs the reader that Christian principles are the means of escaping the castration of death, but the strength of this discourse depends upon the reader's prior identification with Richardson's ideals (S1) and the value system (S2) which promotes and enforces those ideals. The strength of a reader's belief in this system is a key to his/her response. If the reader questions, for example, the word of the moral discourse which promises a heavenly existence after death, the fantasy of a kingdom in paradise seems less appealing than a fantasy of male power on earth.

The novel begins by fracturing paternal authority, and, having questioned the earthly patriarchal power of Clarissa's parents, Richardson's primary discourse attempts to substitute the power of a heavenly patriarch to enforce his moral. In effect, the reader is interpellated away from one father's master discourse to the position of the hysteric, then offered the master discourse of another father to relieve the hysteric's ($'s) "experience of alienation, suppression, and exclusion."[52] As the reaction of readers like Godwin and Lady Bradshaigh indicates, the power of the moral discourse is manifested unevenly. Replacing one father with another creates the possibility of ambiguous results. When Clarissa confuses Lovelace by writing of her impending death, "I am setting out with all diligence for my father's house" (IV 157), his misunderstanding of which

129

father she means echoes the reader's confusion in knowing which father (paternal discourse) to believe. The fathers in the male hierarchy become muddled. Furthermore, if the earthly father's word can be questioned, the word of the patriarchal moral discourse of the earthly Richardson can also be debated.

Lovelace, on the other hand, represents the voice outside of the patriarchy, but he remains a male voice. He creates his own masculinity through his ingenuity and his violence although, symbolically and literally, he has no father. To Lovelace, Clarissa's father's authority is "imaginary" (I 179) and the patriarchal figure of Lord M is a "stupid peer" (II 467). While other men attempt in Lovelace's view to sneak into sin "for fear of detection" (III 389), he acts openly to fulfill what he says all men desire: "Were every rake, nay, were every man, to sit down, as I do, and write all that enters into his head or into his heart, and to accuse himself with equal freedom and truth, what an army of miscreants should I have to keep me in countenance!" (II 492). In Lovelace's terms, he only voices honestly the desires which all men experience.

Unable to rely on the patriarchal system to supply a male identity, Lovelace creates his own hierarchy from his own form of maleness. He stands alone as a man without the support of the system. In order to know that he is recognized as a man, however, he must have the acknowledgment of his masculinity from the men and women he meets. Belford symbolically supplies him with a mirror from which he sees his own magnified reflection. Lovelace desires Belford's "loyalty and love" (I 170), and even though the reformed Belford eventually "rave[s]" at him and calls him "hardened" (IV 133), Lovelace needs him to "proceed with [his] communications" (IV 440). In fact, after making this request in a letter full of remorse, Lovelace has a change of heart and writes an letter which reproduces his earlier arrogance and demands back the previous letter. Even with the significant change in tone, however, Lovelace will "repeat [his] desire" for Belford to "write to me as usual" (IV 444). No matter what mood Lovelace expresses or what Belford's reaction to him may be, Lovelace needs him in order to have a place in this imaginary masculine hierarchy. Even in his final letter to Belford he boasts that "no man . . . has a steadier hand or eye than I have" (IV 526) and that Morden will "take his life or his death at my hands before eleven to-morrow morning" (IV 527). Lovelace's letters to Belford provide him with the opportunity to voice his male authority and to define his position in relation to other men.

At the same time, Lovelace also establishes his maleness by his ability to use and control women. When he succeeds in outwitting Clarissa and inducing her to flee with him, he brags to Belford, "I look down upon everybody now" (I 515), and this moment marks the pinnacle of his masculine power in the novel. In spite of all his manipulative efforts, he will fail to seduce Clarissa, and his rape of Clarissa will punctuate this failure of seduction, the failure of his particular form of masculinity. In this way, his need to have Clarissa is tied directly to his masculine position. "And were I now to lose her," he writes to Belford, "how unworthy should I be to be the prince and leader of such a confraternity as ours!--how unable to look up among men! or to show my face among women!" (II 18). Clarissa, as a woman, provides a gauge against which Lovelace's masculinity can be measured. When he falls short of this "best of women," he proves himself less than the best of men. Without his identity as "king of the rakes," he is nothing, so when he loses control over Clarissa, his confederates who have Clarissa jailed without his knowledge, and his own sanity as he becomes delirious (IV 377), he forfeits his masculinity.

Unlike Sir Charles Grandison, therefore, Lovelace cannot, in the end, retain his male superiority by a union with the ultimate female. What he can claim prior to his fall, however, is an unequaled phallic power of his own creation. While Sir Charles's authority is linked to his hereditary position (he is, after all, _Sir_ Charles) and is presented as unquestioned, Lovelace continually works to control others with his intelligence, good looks, and violent nature. While Sir Charles retains his virtue by being artless and naïve, he also plays a more passive, or feminine, role. Lovelace acts. Although his libertine usage of women masks an attempt to avoid death and castration, he acts on what he believes will give him pleasure and defines his own desire. Furthermore, his interpretation of male desire is not contradicted by the text. Other men would be Lovelace, if they could, but he can do what other men cannot. As Anna Howe writes to Clarissa, even Hickman "would be as saucy as your Lovelace, if he dared. He has not half the arrogant bravery of the other, and can better hide his horns; that's all" (I 340). Richardson presents heterosexual male desire in order to demonstrate the importance of repressing that desire, but the fantasy of unlimited sexual pleasure that Lovelace pursues is an attractive one for readers as well as for libertines.

What emerges from Lovelace's discourse is a view of the world as a testing ground for masculinity. Men do not prove themselves to be men by following a set of rules and accepting a predetermined position in the patriarchy. Instead, life is a constant showdown where male qualities get evaluated by other men and women. In doing so, men establish friendships and animosities with men based upon their relative strengths and weaknesses, and they subordinate women, who function as objects by which a man's masculinity can be measured. Although Richardson intends otherwise, the character of Lovelace provides a model of masculinity which relates both to male desire and to survival in a competitive male world. If Richardson's "method of investigating femininity tends to call masculinity into question,"[53] then the answer to that question of masculinity may be the behavior of his villain. Unable to retire to the country like Sir Charles, Belford, or Hickman, readers might be seduced (in spite of Richardson's efforts) by Lovelace, a man who follows his "own imperial will and pleasure" (I 516).

While Richardson's novels may have influenced the direction of sexuality in the eighteenth century, as Eagleton and Eric Trudgill have suggested,[54] they also present the possibility of masculinities as varied as the behaviors of Lovelace and Grandison. Later, when these masculinities respectively reappear in the form of Gothic villains like Horace Walpole's Manfred in The Castle of Otranto and sentimental heroes like Henry MacKensie's Harley in The Man of Feeling, the ambiguous results of Richardson's project for promoting a more virtuous maleness become apparent. If his "representation of women, female bodies, and femininity, which appears so often to be the focus of the texts, at times seems partly intended to cover for an investigation of men, male bodies, and masculinity,"[55] this investigation reveals a male sexuality in search of an authority, but Richardson's dilemma is that this authority can be read as much in the manipulative actions of Lovelace as the benevolent character of Grandison. Subsequently, readers may, like Godwin, desire to be Lovelace instead of Grandison, and they may also be attracted to those novels which present such villainous predatory males every bit as much as they are to those novels which portray the male as a master of sentiment and compassion. In both cases, the male is the center of the action because he is superior to the others; however, in the case of a Lovelace or a Gothic villain, male sexuality is especially individualistic or narcissistic because it does not depend on social approval, but creates itself in spite of and often contrary to societal sanctions.

Just as Richardson's <u>Clarissa</u> promoted a moral discourse, later Gothic novels ostensibly urged compliance with social norms and discouraged these anti-social and even demonic qualities of the villain; however, readers may have seen aspects of this character as important to survival in a more urban, industrialized, competitive, and male world where order and justice are suspect. In the Gothic, the larger symbols of patriarchal authority like the Church, the Inquisition, or those who enforce the law are as likely to punish the innocent as the guilty. To a certain degree, the Gothic villain, like Lovelace, outwits authority and wages a solitary war in pursuit of his own pleasure against the civilization that would limit that pleasure. The Gothic villain, in much the same way as Lovelace, triumphs only temporarily, but his triumph disregards societal rules and often shows him to be more in control and more actively successful than other characters. His sexuality, in other words, seemingly possesses a power that other masculinities lack, and he proves this power through his resistance and opposition to others.

In their competitive environment, Gothic villains commit heinous social crimes, like murder and incest, almost as a clear signal to readers that these men are totally depraved and should not be used as models of conduct. However, the nature of the masculinity of these villains, represented in their aggressiveness and by their ability to conquer and control, marks them as the most "manly" men in the male universe. While no one believes these male figures were meant to be the prototypes for masculine behavior, readers can see in these characters the means to the fulfillment of desires which the other characters do not possess. As a genre, the novel introduced characters whose individuality required a unique solution that often privileged the individual at the expense of an earlier authority,[56] and most writers, including Defoe and Fielding in addition to Richardson, created characters who struggled against an archaic set of rules which delayed or prevented their happiness. In the Gothic novel, the examination of this struggle broadens rather than disappears. Social changes and the inevitable, accompanying transformations in female/male relations placed an increasing importance on gender identities toward the end of the eighteenth century; consequently, readers enjoyed novels that offered representations of potential sexual alternatives; however, no doubt contrary to Richardson's wishes, readers continued to be able to reject and select, consciously and unconsciously, those images and fantasies which attracted and repulsed them.

Notes

[1]Henry Mackensie, <u>The Man of Feeling</u> (London: Oxford UP, 1967) 82.

[2]Margaret Anne Doody, <u>A Natural Passion: A Study of the Novels of Samuel Richardson</u> (Oxford: Clarendon P, 1974) 18.

[3]Doody 24.

[4]Much has been made of the difference between the male and female Gothic with their respective emphases on the villain and the tormented heroine. Jacqueline Howard in a chapter of her book <u>Reading Gothic Fiction: A Bakhtinian Approach</u> (Oxford: Clarendon P, 1994) entitled "Women and the Gothic," 53-105, attempts to offer a balanced approach to this topic. Howard notes how this separation of gender within the genre has almost unquestioned acceptance from critics. For an example of recent criticism which addresses the Gothic's gender split, see Susan Wolstenholme, preface, <u>Gothic (Re)Visions: Writing Women as Readers</u> (Albany: SUNY P, 1993), xi; see also George Haggerty's discussion of the Female Gothic in "The Gothic Novel, 1764-1824," <u>The Columbia History of the British Novel</u>, ed. John Richetti (New York: Columbia UP, 1994) 223-232.

[5]The Gothic debt to Richardson is a commonplace; for an example of how Richardson's work can be seen to influence the Gothic see Devendra Varma, <u>The Gothic Flame</u> (New York: Russell, 1966) or examine the entries indexed in Frederick S. Frank's bibliographic guide <u>The First Gothics: A Critical Guide to the English Gothic Novel</u> (New York: Garland, 1987).

[6]Doody 149.

[7]Frederick S. Frank, preface, <u>The First Gothics: A Critical Guide to the English Gothic Novel</u> (New York: Garland, 1987) xxv.

[8]William Wordsworth, <u>The Prose Works of William Wordsworth</u>, ed. W. J. B. Owen and Jane Worthington Smyser, Vol. 1, (Oxford: Clarendon, 1974) 128:

> ... a multitude of causes unknown to former times are now acting with a combined force to blunt the discriminating powers of the mind, and unfitting it for all voluntary exertion to reduce it to a state of almost savage torpor. The most effective of these causes are the great national events which are daily taking place, and the encreasing accumulation of men in cities, where the uniformity of their occupations produces a craving for extraordinary incident which the rapid communication of intelligence hourly gratifies. To this tendency of life and manners the literature and theatrical exhibitions of the country have conformed themselves. The invaluable works of our elder writers, I had almost said the works of Shakespear and Milton, are driven into neglect by frantic novels, sickly and stupid German Tragedies, and deluges of idle and extravagant stories in verse.

[9]Elizabeth Kraft, "Public Nurturance and Private Civility: The Transposition of Values in Eighteenth-Century Fiction," <u>Studies in Eighteenth-Century Culture</u>, eds. Patricia B. Craddock and Carla H. Hay, vol. 22 (East Lansing, MI: Colleagues P, 1992) 181-193.

[10]William Godwin, <u>Caleb Williams</u> or <u>Things as They Are</u> (New York: Holt, Rinehart & Winston,1965).

[11]Terry Eagleton, <u>The Rape of Clarissa</u> (Minneapolis: U of Minn P, 1982) 96.

[12]Eric Trudgill, <u>Madonnas and Magdalens: The Origins and Development of Victorian Sexual Attitudes</u> (New York: Holmes & Meier, 1976) 160.

[13]Eagleton 97.

[14]Samuel Richardson, <u>The History of Sir Charles Grandison</u>, ed. Jocelyn Harris, vol. I (London: Oxford, 1972) 14.

[15]Doody 257.

[16]Tom Keymer, <u>Richardson's Clarissa and the Eighteenth-Century Reader</u> (Cambridge: Cambridge UP, 1992) 196.

[17]Jocelyn Harris, introduction, <u>The History of Sir Charles Grandison</u>, vol. I, by Samuel Richardson (London: Oxford, 1972) xix.

[18]Tassie Gwilliam, <u>Samuel Richardson's Fictions of Gender</u> (Stanford: Stanford UP, 1993) points out how Sir Charles is the "offspring of a 'rake' and an 'angel' who bear strong resemblances to Lovelace and Clarissa," 112.

[19]Doody 274.

[20]Richardson, <u>SCG</u> I, 55.

[21]Richardson, <u>SCG</u> I, 134.

[22]Richardson, <u>SCG</u> I, 140.

[23]Gwilliam 122-133 discusses the theme of castration in <u>Grandison</u>; I would suggest that the reason that the other males are unmanned is because this is the only way for Richardson to "masculate" his otherwise passive hero.

[24]Doody 274.

[25]Tom Keymer, "Clarissa's Death, <u>Clarissa</u>'s Sale, and the Text of the Second Edition," <u>Review of English Studies</u> 45 (1994) 389.

[26]Sylvia Kasey Marks, <u>Sir Charles Grandison: The Compleat Conduct Book</u> (Lewisburg: Bucknell UP, 1986) 13.

[27]Doody 274.

[28]Keymer, "Clarissa's Death," 395.

[29]Keymer, "Clarissa's Death," 395

[30]Samuel Richardson, <u>Clarissa</u>, 4 vols. (London: Dent, 1985); all subsequent references will be made to this same edition.

[31]Betty A. Schellenberg, "Using 'Femalities' to 'Make Fine Men': Richardson's <u>Sir Charles Grandison</u> and the Feminization of Narrative," <u>Studies in English Literature, 1500-1800</u> 34 (1994): note 614.

[32]Richardson, qtd. in Marks 54

[33]Richardson, <u>SCG</u> I, 3.

[34]Richardson, <u>SCG</u> I, 4.

[35]Keymer, <u>Richardson's Clarissa</u>, 196

[36]Keymer, <u>Richardson's Clarissa</u>, 196.

[37]Schellenberg 613

[38]Mark Bracher, <u>Lacan, Discourse, and Social Change: A Psychoanalytic Cultural Criticism</u> (Ithaca: Cornell UP, 1993) 53.

[39]Bracher 53

[40]Bracher 35.

[41]Bracher 46.

[42]Doody 124.

[43]Doody 125.

[44]Lois E. Bueler, <u>Clarissa's Plots</u> (Newark: U of Del P, 1994) 109.

[45]Bracher 48.

[46]Bracher 21.

[47]Samuel Richardson, author's preface, <u>Clarissa,</u> vol 1 (London: Dent, 1985) xiv.

[48]Doody 166.

[49]Doody 151-187.

[50]Richardson, preface, <u>Clarissa</u>, xv.

[51]Patricia Meyer Spacks, <u>Desire and Truth: Functions of Plot in Eighteenth-Century English Novels</u> (Chicago: U of Chicago P, 1990) 57.

[52]Bracher 54.

[53]Gwilliam 6.

[54]Eagleton 96-97, and Trudgill 160.

[55]Gwilliam 9.

[56]Ian Watt, <u>The Rise of the Novel: Studies in Defoe, Richardson and Fielding</u> (Berkeley: U of Cal P, 1964) puts forth what is now a well-established connection between the rise of the novel and the growing importance of the individual.

CHAPTER V

WALPOLE AND GOTHIC MASCULINITY

The Mysterious Mother is the most disgusting, detestable, vile composition that ever came from the hand of man. No one with a spark of true manliness, of which Horace Walpole had none, could have written it.

Samuel Taylor Coleridge[1]

Coleridge's revulsion with Horace Walpole's unproduced Gothic drama The Mysterious Mother not only provides an example of the often negative critical reaction to all Gothic works and Gothic writers, but also suggests the importance of sexual identity in the history of literary authority. In recent years, feminist critics have properly called attention to the unfair, gender-based exclusion of female writers from what had been a male dominated canon; however, this critical reexamination has not gone far enough. Male Gothic writers and their works, often categorized as aberrant or perverse by critics like Coleridge, should be reconsidered apart from such stigmatizing assessments.

If sexuality was restructured or redirected during the eighteenth century,[2] then the traditional division between the canonical greats (Richardson, Fielding, and Smollett) who have been used as a literary and sexually normative standard and the male Gothic writers (Walpole, Lewis, and Godwin) who have generally been presented as sexually and literarily aberrant may have larger implications. The continued tendency for critics like George Haggerty, who suggests that "male homosexuality is one of the secrets of Gothic fiction,"[3] to classify Gothic novelists as well as novels as somehow sexually different, anti-societal, or revolutionary perhaps demonstrates how closely linked these impulses toward gender and genre classifications are. While Haggerty's work is interesting in its emphasis on the sexual nature of the Gothic novel, his intention of finding a sexual difference between male Gothic novelists and other male novelists functions in the same way as Coleridge's remarks. In both instances, the Gothic novelist is viewed as sexually abnormal and, consequently, the Gothic work he produced can be discounted as the product of an aberrant fantasy.

This emphasis on an "other" sexuality for Gothic novelists and novels, however, overlooks the possibility that readers found in these novels a masculinity which they could identify with, which engaged their desires, and which was not necessarily bounded by societal limitations. Instead of attempting to categorize these texts and their authors, as has always been done, I believe that a more useful approach reexamines each text for the purpose of understanding its possible interpellative impact on its many readers. The value of this approach, in my opinion, is that it focuses on the various masculine representations found in the text and avoids those conclusions which demand a separateness for the Gothic novel and a judgment of the sexual nature of the text or the author.

Because the Gothic villain, or antihero, proved to be so popular, he needs to be better understood. As "an overreacher seeking power, pleasure, even godhood," the Gothic villain may suffer from extreme "egotism and monomania"[4] and, consequently, represent a different masculinity than Tom Jones, Robinson Crusoe, or Humphrey Clinker, but it is his character which makes the most popular Gothic novels interesting. This is especially true for the male Gothic writers, but even the heroine-centered novels of Ann Radcliffe have memorable villains like Montoni (<u>The Mysteries of Udolpho</u>) and Schedoni (<u>The Italian</u>). It is not enough to assume that, because these representations of masculinity display clear moral flaws and anti-social characteristics, the reader disregards the manner in which these characters "creat[e] or recreat[e] their own identities" and realize their desires "through the efforts of their own wills."[5] On the contrary, the continued popularity of the Gothic novel in spite of widespread critical disapproval indicates that readers may have found something in these books and in these villains which related to the readers' own fantasies of power or sexuality or anti-social behavior. The "double-faced reception" of <u>The Castle of Otranto,</u> which was "a hit with the public" while receiving "disapprobation from the critics,"[6] was indicative of the response that would follow the publication of Godwin's <u>Caleb Williams</u>, and Lewis's <u>The Monk</u>. In reexamining the Gothic, therefore, perhaps it is time we put aside the critical heritage that has shunned or demeaned these books and, instead, try to recreate those qualities that readers found so attractive. Within these texts whose plots formulaically take place amid ruined castles, labyrinthine dungeons, and haunted scenery, there is something which so appealed to readers that between 4,500 to 5,000 Gothic novels were published before 1820.[7] Perhaps the forbidden sexuality generally represented by the villain was more interesting and recognizable to readers than critics would like to admit.

William Patrick Day has said that the pleasure of reading a Gothic text depends upon the reader's ability to position himself or herself at a distance from the text as a voyeur who safely explores the limits of both fear and desire;[8] however, what concerns me is not the reader's position as voyeur, which seems to be a much bigger question involving anything read or viewed, but the nature of those desires which lead the reader to those fears and desires generated by popular genres like the Gothic novel. The appeal in the eighteenth century of the narcissistic villain suggests that readers enjoyed his displays of masculine power even while they rooted for his demise, and the continued existence of similar masculine types in a number of current horror movies and action films confirms the resiliency of what has become a stock character. If these generally hypermasculine villains involve us in a "sadomasochistic" fantasy and "enthrall"[9] us, then we need to determine what elements in these male characters we identify with and what desires are engaged. By beginning with an analysis of Walpole's Manfred, the "archetype"[10] of the Gothic villain, I hope to show the forces at work in the creation and in the attraction of such characters. As the villain in the first Gothic novel, Manfred provides the blueprint for the evil masculine role which will be followed by the anti-heroes of subsequent Gothic novels. Although Walpole did not possess Richardson's ability to present "delicate shades of character,"[11] he was able to establish the image of the troubled tyrant in the midst of a crumbling and predatory world which would provide future Gothic novelists the starting point for their own more complex creations.

While Walpole has been called "the father" of the Gothic novel,[12] this paternal relationship has been critically associated as much with censure as acclaim. Whether or not this association with an "audacious genre which [until recently] had long been regarded . . . as an inconsequential and superficial literary tradition"[13] has helped or harmed his reputation as a writer of fiction remains undetermined; nevertheless, his novel, The Castle of Otranto, has enjoyed repeated publication, and since the first "twenty-one editions of the book in the eighteenth century,"[14] "Otranto has never slipped from sight."[15] Although the foremost Walpolean scholar, Wilmarth S.

Lewis, argues that Otranto's continual reprinting is owing to its continued popularity,[16] the majority of critical opinion seems to focus on the text's historical significance and ignores the text itself. Paradoxically, a book which has appeared in more than 150 editions[17] has "received relatively scant attention"[18] from critics except those discussing the development of the Gothic genre, or sub-genre.[19] Consequently, while much has been made of Manfred's status as the original Gothic villain in Otranto, little light has been shed on the importance of Walpole's presentation of this prototypical male character. Nevertheless, Manfred represents a new type of male character which will inevitably take the form of the more critically renowned Byronic hero.[20]

Even though Walpole's often discussed parentage of the Gothic sub-genre begins with his construction of "the first Gothic castle on the literary landscape of 1764"[21] and extends to his subtitle of A Gothic Story (which forever classified this species of romance) attached to the second edition of Otranto, his most lasting contribution to the greater genre of the novel may be this Gothic villain Manfred, who pursues his desire beyond societal rules and in spite of continuing catastrophic consequences. Like Lovelace, Manfred is a male character whose sexual presence dictates the action of a novel and whose potential to possess a forbidden pleasure (*jouissance*) marks him as someone in possession of phallic power. In Manfred, however, Walpole's fascination with Sophocles' Oedipus Rex and, as Betsy Harfst and Martin Kallich have attempted to elucidate, Walpole's own conscious and unconscious concerns about parricide, incest, and castration[22] combine to create a male character who not only seeks phallic immortality through his union with a woman, but who also struggles against a fate which he has inherited from his father. In spite of Harfst's and Kallich's efforts, Walpole's own

Oedipal conflict seems less obvious and less important in <u>Otranto</u> than the problems of the text's main character, which may or may not be linked to the psychological make-up of the author. Nevertheless, their critical commentary serves to point out the often overlooked psychological complexity of a character that has otherwise been considered what Kallich himself labels as "stock."[23]

Rather than a stock character, Manfred is an ambiguous original, a man caught between the overwhelming desire for regeneration and the control of his kingdom and a prophetic awareness of the inevitable annihilation of his progeny due to the treachery of his grandfather. Instead of seeking to create a new masculinity based on an individual authority like Lovelace, Manfred tries to install himself as patriarch without a legitimate claim to the throne. Therefore, while he shows Lovelace's refusal to acknowledge castration (literally, the cutting off of his lineage) and death, he retains a desire to reestablish the hierarchy that Lovelace denounces. Simultaneously, Manfred is the son who wishes to be the father, and he is also the son whose (grand)father's actions have condemned him. Ultimately, he would deny castration by assuming the position of the primal father who has access to all of the women; however, he is frustrated in his efforts because he is not the father, but a son who must eventually face his own powerlessness. As the man who would be king, Walpole's villainous creation is a reflection of an author and perhaps an age attempting to reconcile a desire for order and authority with a recognition of the abuses of absolute power.

Walpole's own relationship with his father, the powerful British Prime Minister Sir Robert Walpole, may have influenced his characterization of this son fighting to retain a power his family deceitfully claimed. Lewis describes Horace as demonstrating both "outward loyalty"[24] and "latent hostility"[25] toward his father, and these ambiguous feelings appear in the character of Manfred who owes his kingdom to his grandfather but who is punished for his grandfather's crimes. However, Manfred is also the creation of a man who longed for a simpler time and could write to his friend George Montagu:

> I almost think there is no wisdom comparable to that of exchang-
> ing what is called the realities of life for dreams. Old castles, old
> pictures, old histories, and the babble of old people make one live
> back into centuries, that cannot disappoint one. One holds fast
> and surely what is past. The dead have exhausted their power of
> deceiving....[26]

Walpole's words describe a yearning for that completeness which is represented in psychoanalytic theory by the phallus in the person of the missing father. In turn, the Gothic novel, in Walpole's hands, is the ground upon which the past is rebuilt and the mythical primal father restored to power; furthermore, while Manfred represents the man who would rule this fantastical land, he also demonstrates the failure of a modern man (he is after all, "Man"-fred and not the immortalized King Alfred) to attain the phallic authority which is available to those in the past who are dead and, therefore, unchang-ing and monolithic. In short, death provides a phallic completeness which can be pursued in life but never attained. Consequently, even while the past represents the unchangeable, it is also a reminder of our own mortality for it is only in death that we become undisap-pointing, stable beings. Manfred's rule, therefore, is an impossibility because he is not the father, but a castrated son unable to perpetuate himself and subject to the limitations of mortality.

Manfred's attempt at perpetuating himself through his lineage only brings him face to face with his own radical incompleteness. For Manfred, this means that his burden is the knowledge of his own castration, or the knowledge that he cannot be the Father, the possessor of phallic power and, in Freud's terms, the mythical primal father. Walpole's expressed moral in the Preface to <u>Otranto</u>, "that the sins of fathers are visited on their children to the third and fourth generation" (5), indicates both a preoccupation with the consequences of misplaced paternal power and a desire for a return to the order established by the missing primal father. Before social stability in <u>Otranto</u> can be established, however, the correct father must be discovered. Manfred would believe himself to be the primal father as he initially lays claim to an immortality and an unrestrained power which marks him as a phallic authority. Nevertheless, he loses his son and, subsequently, his principality to the supernatural vengeance of the dead Alfonso the Good, the actual missing father, who, in turn, restores the principality to his issue by posthumously revealing his previously unknown fatherhood. At the same time that the antagonistic claims of these two fathers provide the story's primary conflict, Frederic, Isabella's father, and Father Jerome, the holy father and Theodore's father, also challenge Manfred's authority. The right to control the real estate, the women and children, and the future of Otranto beyond one's lifetime depends upon which father proves superior; however, final phallic authority resides only in the missing father.

In <u>Otranto</u>, Walpole confronts the same dilemma which Richardson faces in <u>Clarissa</u>: If the earthly father is suspect, whose word is to be believed? While Richardson solves this problem by employing the discourse of Christian principles and sending Clarissa to her "father's" house in heaven, Walpole is not so easily able to resolve this conflict and his ending reflects his own ambiguous spirituality. Although he "accepted the Christian ethic," Walpole "rejected the supernatural doctrines of Christianity,"[27] and his story's uneven moral shares this ambiguity. Manfred clearly is an illegitimate father figure, and he loses his kingdom to the indiscriminate and apparently limitless power of Alfonso the Good; however, the ending, while restoring order, leaves little reason for the earthly survivors to rejoice. While Manfred as the father tyrannizes over the other characters, Manfred as the son is punished for his father's transgressions; at the same time, while Alfonso the Good triumphs with the return of his progeny to the throne, his descendant Theodore loses the woman he loves and inherits a kingdom in ruins.

Initially, however, Manfred resembles Freud's primal father, the dominant male who has access to all the women. He appears to be monolithic and solitary. As a usurper, he rules Otranto while remaining symbolically outside of the system. He seemingly holds the secret to unknown and forbidden pleasures, having had an arguably incestuous marriage (49) with Hippolita and pursuing a symbolically incestuous relationship with Isabella, his proposed daughter-in-law. Manfred appears to be both the source of law and outside of the law. From his phallic perspective, the female exists only as an object of male desire or as an article of property. In fact, Hippolita and Isabella have importance only as a previous or potential female sexual object because of their inability or ability to bear him a son. Marriage for Manfred is a property transaction and Isabella's marriage is a means for her "charms" to be "disposed of" (22). The emphasis on male lineage in <u>Otranto</u> is so pervasive that Manfred rejects that line of descendants which would extend from his daughter Matilda. Instead, he is obsessed with creating a male heir and preserving his claim to Otranto in the name of his family. As the supreme male, he controls all the females and challenges or commands the other males. No man conquers him nor seems capable of doing so. Frederic, a "weak prince" (92), threatens him, but holds "little hope of dispossessing [him] by force" (92). In the end, Manfred is not forced to abdicate his title but does so by his own will and, in the process, permits Theodore, the grandson of Alfonso, to rule. Theodore does not take power from Manfred; Manfred cedes the power to Theodore.

Provided with almost unlimited power over the other characters of the novel, Manfred receives his only physical opposition from supernatural forces that drop a gigantic helmet on his son and involve themselves in enough scenes of terror to help to motivate his repentance. While he reacts to this series of apparitions, which include his grandfather Roderic's ghost emerging from a portrait in his presence, the primary impetus for his action and the action of the novel remains his desire to reproduce himself in the image of a son. Even with all of his power, he is not immortal, and it is his knowledge of this mortality which motivates him to act in a villainous fashion by casting aside Hippolita and pursuing Isabella. In spite of, or, perhaps, in direct confrontation with, a prophecy which foretells the end of his lineage and that immortality represented by the control of Otranto through future generations, Manfred fights the castrating forces which would "cut-off" his family's rule and force him to acknowledge his own incompleteness. His brazen pursuit of Isabella so that he might have a male heir is impelled by a desire that surpasses an attempt to continue the family's reign in Otranto and equates possessing her and the prospective male offspring with an implied "real" immortality.

When Conrad, Manfred's son, dies at the beginning of Otranto, his position as the missing male heir immediately represents this lost immortality, the lost object or the object a, to Manfred. For the remainder of the novel, Manfred will seek this object a, the object of desire. He responds to his son's death with indifference toward his "disfigured corpse" (17), but immediately takes action to create a replacement. "[T]he first sounds that dropped from Manfred's lips were, 'Take care of the lady Isabella' " (17). From this point on, Walpole, through his principal character Manfred, will metonymi-cally link Isabella's person, Isabella's birthright, the creation of a male heir, and Manfred's own rule over Otranto, and each of these ideas will, in turn, metaphorically represent the lost object of Manfred's immortality. Manfred's expression of desire, "I want Isabella" (34), embodies all of these connected ideas and simplifies for the reader an otherwise confusing motive. If he pursues Isabella "to unite the claims" (59) of his house with hers, then why does he do so in such a desperate manner, especially when he is "too powerful for the house of Vicenza to dispossess" (59)? Why does Manfred not, as Father Jerome fears, direct himself "to some other object" (49) which could bear him the son he desires? Why is his need so urgent when the possibility remains, as Frederic considers, "that no issue might succeed from the union" (92) of Manfred and Isabella? The prophecy that Manfred's family "should reign in Otranto until the rightful owner should be grown too large to inhabit the castle, and as long as issue-male from Ricardo's [Manfred's grandfather's] loins should remain to enjoy it" (109) does not answer these questions or clarify Manfred's ambiguous motivation. The prophecy actually makes time and the woman who bears the son irrelevant. These contradictions are unimportant because the idea expressed in the statement, "I want Isabella," both confuses and conflates them. All that is made apparent is that Manfred desires and what he desires is represented by Isabella.

Therefore, while Walpole provides political reasons for Manfred's pursuit of Isabella, the main impetus for the action is heterosexual male fantasy ($\$ <> \underline{a}$). By definition, Manfred is the split subject ($\$$) in relation to the woman Isabella, the object of desire ($\underline{a}$). In this fantasy, if Manfred possesses Isabella, he becomes whole (uncastrated), and, in <u>Otranto</u>, male possession of a woman implies physical possession. After Manfred informs Isabella of his intention to marry her, she flees him to "avoid the impetuosity of his passions"(24) and "for that night at least avoid his odious purpose" (25).

Furthermore, male desire is seen as uncontrollable and equated with violence. When she fears that "her rash flight" has "exposed her to his rage in a place where her cries were not likely to draw any body to her assistance" (25), she acknowledges that Manfred's desire for her will result in a form of violence that implies rape. In this way, the phallic man in pursuit of the object of his desires is viewed as likely to use whatever means available to gain satisfaction. Although rape, in Otranto, is not stated but only implied as another example of Manfred's tyranny or the abuse of his male power, his ability to take what he wants through a "rage" that suggests rape proves this power and is tied directly to his masculinity. Subsequently, his failure to catch and rape Isabella marks the beginning of his decline in power and his loss of position as the dominant male.

Unlike Richardson, who offers in Clarissa competing discourses which are intended to direct the reader toward what Richardson saw as the superior discourse of Christian principles, Walpole primarily presents the master discourse of a patriarchal property struggle and the corresponding fantasy of male completion through possession of the body of the desired female. In other words, Manfred's discourse simultaneously uses the master signifiers which describe the importance of "preserving my race" (24) and reveals the fantasy operating beneath this master discourse. In this equation,[28]

$$\frac{S1 \dashrightarrow S2}{\$ \qquad \underline{a}}$$

S1 ---> S2 represents the continued dominance of the signifiers which promote an ultimate male authority that hides, or represses, the underlying fantasy of male completeness. This fantasy ($ <> $\underline{a}$) which is embodied (in the Imaginary register) by Manfred's physical pursuit of Isabella is actually his desire for his lost immortality, the lack-of-being that is denied by an ego ideal which conceals the search for an impossible lost object $\underline{a}$ by voicing (in the Symbolic register) and physically demonstrating (in the Imaginary register) the desire for an heir. Manfred's ultimate failure does not defeat this discourse since his conqueror Alfonso actually has achieved the totality that Manfred seeks, but instead this failure implies that Manfred's effort is somehow insufficient to the task.

Because Isabella is able to elude "Manfred's hated bed" (88), he loses both his principality and his masculinity. Having established her as necessary for his own masculine completion, he must possess her (even by killing her) or admit castration. In Otranto, possessing the woman that one desires is an important indication of masculinity, and one forfeits at least part of that masculinity by losing the woman, the object of desire. Frederic negotiates for Matilda and would possess her until the appearance of a skeleton convinces him to desire otherwise. Theodore can have either Matilda or Isabella, who both desire him. He chooses Matilda, but because she dies, eventually accepts Isabella as a lesser substitute. Even Alfonso the Good has had the choice of tempting the "fair virgin named Victoria" to "forbidden pleasures"(110) or marrying her first. Since he is "good," the socially stabilizing element in the novel requires that he marries her, but the choice remains his. While Manfred's methods may be questioned, the male power that he asserts is not. Hippolita remarks that the male hierarchy, "heaven, our fathers, and our husbands" (88), should decide for females the disposition of their bodies, and the text supports this proposition.

At stake for Manfred, then, is not only his position in Otranto but his signification as a man. Except for the apparitions, no one threatens his rule and even the prophecy does not suggest that he could be deposed in his lifetime. However, once he has established Isabella as the object of his desire, he must either possess her or lose his masculinity. Her significance to Manfred relates entirely to his success in maintaining his male authority. When he draws his dagger to kill her, he does so because of what she represents in terms of his relationships with other men. At the time of his attack, he is "enraged at her father" (104) and believes she is arranging to marry Theodore. In other words, though Isabella has a stated aesthetic value because of her "beauty" and "charms" (22), her real importance to Manfred coincides directly to his position in the male hierarchy. He does not need to marry her to affirm that position. If he rapes or kills her, he signifies his superiority to the other males. Ironically, he mistakenly kills Matilda instead of Isabella and thereby cuts off his own bloodlines as well as his opportunity to exchange his daughter with Frederic for Isabella. In effect, he symbolically castrates himself.

The moral ending to the story, therefore, reduces Manfred to a mortal being by cutting off his hopes of symbolic immortality. His reply to Hippolita after the walls of his castle are thrown down, "My heart at last is open to thy devout admonitions" (108), indicates that he finally understands his own mortality and that the only real immortality is a heavenly one. In spite of his earthly "power and wealth" (96), even Manfred must succumb to the "will of heaven" (109). Although this lesson seems apparent to the reader from the beginning when a gigantic helmet falls from the sky, Manfred's reliance on his passions and power to accomplish what even "divine and human laws forbid" (88) prevents him from recognizing the obvious. Like Frederic, "the portents that had alarmed him were forgotten in his desires" (103), but, unlike Frederic, Manfred's desires are not simply for possession of an attractive female. While Frederic concedes his immediate claim to Otranto by agreeing to the trade of daughters as wives, Manfred works singularly for the purpose of securing his claim in perpetuity. He consistently focuses his efforts on obtaining the lost object of his immortality, which Isabella represents.

Manfred's passionate refusal to accept his mortal consequences functions, for the reader, as an expression of the drives as they are opposed by the law of the Symbolic order. As the father possessing phallic power, Manfred appears to be capable of escaping symbolic castration and transcending the law. As Isabella's "father in law" (23), he disregards the societal rules which consider their relationship incestuous. In addition, he has already broken the incest taboo in his marriage to Hippolita who "is related to [him] in the fourth degree" (49). Manfred ignores the law and seemingly has access to a *jouissance* outside of the system. Consequently, until his downfall, he occupies "the position of the mythical father of Freud's primal horde, the one exception to the restriction of *jouissance*."[29] Manfred's eventual symbolic castration, however, reminds the reader of the inability of the drives to attain wholeness or, in other words, to regain the bliss that has been lost by assimilation into the Symbolic order. With Manfred's retirement to the convent on the final page, Walpole directs both his character and the reader toward heaven, the only location where completion can presumably be found.

This opposition between the drives and the Symbolic order is reinforced in the Imaginary register by the repeated images of castration found in the fragmented bodies which appear supernaturally in the form of the helmet (17), the foot and leg (33), the hand (98), and the skeleton (103). Since the source of these phenomena is the Symbolic Other in the form of saint Nicholas (sic) or Alfonso the Good or some other unidentified divine power, the message to Manfred is to recognize the word of this Other and his own castration. While Manfred fails to heed this message, readers experience these images and their meaning as a threat to their identity in the

Imaginary register. Instead of denying castration by assuming an identity which includes an image of physical completeness, readers are forced to confront the fractured images of fragmented bodies and the inevitable reality of death. Conrad's violent death and the description of his "bleeding mangled remains" (17) on the third page of the narrative quickly provide a vivid reminder of the reader's physical vulnerability. The description of "the horror of the spectacle . . . [which] took away the prince's speech" (17) informs the reader that he or she has just entered a world outside of symbolic representation where no one is safe. In the images of this world, the reader will not find completeness or security, but will be confronted continually with the fragmented images which threaten his or her image of bodily integrity.

The Gothic novel, in this manner, offers the reader a sublime landscape in which to travel. Against this landscape, the reader feels vulnerable to the greater powers in and possibly outside of nature. The supernatural in Otranto operates to recall the insecurity of the ideal ego upon recognition of those powers outside of itself which it does not possess or control. The act of reading a Gothic novel like Otranto places the reader in a position not only to observe the symbolic castration of the villain but also to recognize his or her own incompleteness or castration. Like Manfred, readers may be cut off from a comfortable belief in their imaginary identity and may have to seek a symbolic substitute. In Otranto, however, no one offers a successful discourse. While Manfred is clearly the focus of the wrath of the Symbolic Other, in the figures of the other characters, the reader also experiences the horrors that appear on the Gothic terrain. The alternative discourses offered by the other males and by the females in the novel do not prevent the repeated images of castration that end only when Otranto is in ruins. The reader, interpellated into the position of the hysteric ($) confronted by castration, has no obvious master discourse to turn to for a resolution in the Symbolic register. Although readers are unlikely to accept Manfred's corrupt and depraved methods of pursuing his fantasy of phallic completion, they may share this fantasy of a pleasure and wholeness outside of language and law and search for a discourse in the novel which will alleviate their anxiety. However, unlike Richardson in Clarissa, Walpole does not offer a strong master discourse of Christian values (S1 --> S2) in opposition to Manfred's discourse of male authority. Instead, Walpole provides the competing discourses of the male characters, who mirror each other in their belief in a superior male authority, and readers eventually must choose a male voice to follow if they wish to resolve the tension created between the unrestrained desires of Manfred and the limiting forces of the Symbolic Other (saint Nicholas, Alfonso and the heavenly powers).

All of the male characters, however, seem driven by the same desire to possess the kingdom and the women in it. The only alternative discourse that opposes this desire for power is presented by Hippolita and Matilda, but this discourse not only fails to resolve the anxiety created by the fragmented images but also supports the overriding message of male supremacy. In denying desire, both female characters accept their subservient position to male authority and have almost no subjectivity whatsoever. "Hippolita's unbounded submission to the will of her lord" (60) is echoed by Matilda who, even after Manfred has inflicted the fatal dagger wound, asks his forgiveness for her accidental disobedience (105). Matilda's one lapse from "filial duty" (68) is to "suffer a passion to enter [her] heart" (88) without parental approval and, as a result, to release Theodore from the black tower. Theodore's freedom, in turn, leads eventually to her death when Manfred mistakes her for Isabella when he hears her talking to Theodore by the tomb of Alfonso. Matilda, who has an "inclination for the cloister" (44), experiences desire and dies because of it. Ironically, the "great saint Nicholas" (39), whom she "pray[s] to for a husband" (39), appears to orchestrate her demise along with all the other catastrophic events when he appears in the clouds at the end. The Symbolic Other in the form of saint Nicholas opposes the desire embodied by Manfred while his most devout followers, Hippolita, whose "soul is set on heaven" (47) and Matilda, promote a discourse of obedience in place of individual desire. Their voice, however, is an ineffective, female voice which influences Manfred only when Matilda lies dying and the male power at the root of her discourse becomes apparent. At this point, when he recognizes his own subservience to a higher authority, he has been castrated and symbolically made feminine himself, thereby recalling his earlier equation of "the whining of priests" with "the shrieks of women" (54). When he finally listens to the discourse of Hippolita, he abandons his principality and, correspondingly, his masculinity.

Therefore, in the same way that Isabella represents the object a of desire, Manfred's castration becomes represented by Hippolita, who urges him to resign (90) and whose inability to have additional children signifies a sterility that connects to her non-sexual position as a "saint" (49). The union of Manfred and Hippolita has been promoted by the story line which continually reminds the reader of Hippolita's "virtue" (49), but the action of the story and the reader's interest in the characters are maintained by Manfred's struggle to have Isabella. Manfred's choice between Hippolita and Isabella is a choice between an embrace of "virtue," or, in other words, the rules put forth by the Symbolic order, and the drives, enacted by the pursuit of individual desire. While the reader understands the moral solution, he or she remains simultaneously attracted and repulsed by the promise of the unknown pleasure of Manfred's union with Isabella. In effect, the reader's own fantasies are evoked by the unwritten possibilities implied by the potential for Manfred to capture Isabella and to get her alone. Manfred's prolonged denial of castration permits these fantasies to continue to operate until the final pages.

When the other male characters are introduced into the plot, they appear capable of providing the voice for male authority which will resolve the conflict between Manfred's desires and the Symbolic Other who haunts the landscape. Theodore seemingly knows the source of the mystery when he identifies the helmet as resembling that of a statue of Alfonso the Good and appears to be the prototypical hero in his defense of Isabella. Jerome has "saint-like virtues" (45) and intercedes with Manfred on behalf of Isabella and Hippolita. Frederic arrives with a cavalcade of attendants, one hundred of whom carry "an enormous sword" (62), the obvious symbol of some great phallic power. Yet, each of these men fails to bring about an adequate resolution. Jerome almost gets his son Theodore beheaded by misleading Manfred and making him jealous. Frederic loses in single combat to Theodore, and his own "scruples" (100) are weak in comparison to his desire for Matilda. Theodore, meanwhile, mistakenly challenges and injures Frederic, then later fails to protect Matilda, who dies at the blade of her father while standing beside Theodore.

Even saint Nicholas and Alfonso the Good deliver ambiguous male messages. Their respective signifiers, "saint" and "good," and their position in the clouds identify them as heavenly sources of a value system which will set things right, but saint Nicholas had accepted "a church and two convents" (109) from Ricardo in return for Ricardo's life and a limited reign in Otranto, and Alfonso extracts vengeance on the innocent Conrad and Matilda. Although the problem of the hereditary claim to Otranto gets solved, the moral message of the novel is unclear. Manfred and Hippolita, though they utilize opposing discourses, suffer the identical fate of losing two children and retiring to a convent. Meanwhile, Theodore's reward for virtuous conduct is to rule a devastated principality and to "forever indulge the melancholy that had taken possession of his soul" (110). While Manfred's fall (castration) eliminates the tension between the drives and the value system of the Symbolic order, the type of male conduct promoted by the Symbolic order remains unclear.

Manfred's two options, "to resign his dominions" or "to press his marriage with Isabella" (95), represent a choice between acceptance of castration or pursuit of desire. If Manfred resigns, he loses his male authority and his masculinity, but if he pursues Isabella, he breaks the law of the Symbolic Other and risks the castration that is threatened by the sequence of apparitions. To be a man, he must challenge the ultimate phallic power possessed by the heavenly agents, Alfonso the Good and saint Nicholas, but such a challenge must finally prove his own insufficiency. While confronting the Symbolic Other, the origin of the value system, is, by definition, morally wrong, Manfred, "prince of Otranto" (15), has no other choice if he wishes to keep his identity. At the same time, therefore, that he commits acts that the reader recognizes as socially unacceptable, Manfred also courageously defends his signification as a "male" and a "prince." Paradoxically, the same actions that make Manfred barbaric or inhuman also operate to secure his masculinity.

Furthermore, though his violent methods threaten Theodore, Isabella, Jerome, Frederic, Matilda and, by interpellative effect, the reader, Manfred's violence is overshadowed by the actions of the Symbolic Other, who provides the primary destructive power in the novel. In order to keep his masculinity, Manfred has no alternative but to meet the savagery that crushes his son with his own "rage." Manfred fails, in part, because his brutality does not succeed. He does not rape Isabella or kill Theodore, two actions which would alter the course of the novel. Because "Manfred was not one of those savage tyrants who wanton in cruelty unprovoked" (30), he does not have Theodore killed in the subterraneous passage, and because he is "struck . . . with terror" (57) at the arrival of Frederic with the gigantic sword, Manfred negotiates with Jerome and spares Theodore's life. Manfred fails to execute Theodore because of his "naturally humane" (30) temper and his fear, two characteristics that operate against his authority and end up costing him his sovereignty. In other words, Manfred loses the principality to Theodore not because he is savage, but because he is not savage enough.

At the same time that Manfred fails to murder Theodore, the Symbolic Other in the form of saint Nicholas and Alfonso kills the innocent Conrad, destroys the castle, and controls the events that lead to the death of the innocent Matilda. The phallic control that Manfred fails to establish is possessed in the end by Alfonso and saint Nicholas, who have the immortality and the unlimited power that Manfred lacks. Their own unrestricted cruelty would appear to make them comparable to Manfred as tyrants; however, because they represent the Law, their actions are moral while Manfred's are not. Theodore's question, "Will heaven visit the innocent for the crimes of the guilty?" (91), is clearly answered in the affirmative, but readers accept this seemingly unjust doctrine because it is decreed by the Symbolic Other in the persons of the heavenly Nicholas and Alfonso. The victory of the Symbolic Other restores order and provides narrative closure. It also ends the conflict between the drives and the Symbolic order that has led to the series of fragmented images and the reader's damaged sense of bodily integrity.

However, Alfonso shows himself to be the superior male and regains Otranto for his progeny only by using more violence than Manfred.

Ostensibly, then, the Law of the Symbolic order is reestablished and social stability is restored at the end of Otranto. This return to order ends the conflict which has created the multiple images of castration and brings the reader back to a position where he or she no longer feels threatened. The marriage of Isabella and Theodore in the final lines unites the two remaining male forces (the families of Frederic and Alfonso) and symbolically provides the completion that the fragmented images and Manfred's struggle for the object of desire have denied and prevented. But, while the ending supplies narrative closure, Walpole's message remains ambiguous. Manfred's desires are no more responsible for the catastrophic events than the Law which seeks to prevent those desires. Furthermore, the novel's interpellative force is generated by the reader's recognition and internalization of the phallic fantasies which motivate Manfred and also lie at the heart of Nicholas and Alfonso's, the Symbolic Other's, power. There is little difference between the behavior of Manfred and that of the Symbolic Other. Though the ending seems to promote obedience to societal standards, the text shows those standards to be arbitrarily chosen by the man in control whose legitimacy is proven by the destruction of his adversary.

In spite of the traditional meaning inherent in the defeat of the villain and the hero's marriage, final symbolic authority is missing from the ending of Otranto. As a result of the struggle among the various fathers (Manfred, Jerome, Frederic, Alfonso, and even the patriarchal figure of saint Nicholas), Theodore, the only character to be represented as a son in the novel, claims the final position of male authority as the "sovereign of Otranto" (106). Because Alfonso is the victorious Father in the struggle for control of Otranto, Theodore inherits the principality. Theodore rules Otranto, but what he gets is a destroyed castle and the right to rule without the woman he desired. In other words, he must abide by the terms dictated by Alfonso, his grandfather. He assumes his masculine position as "prince" (106) at the cost of his object of desire, Matilda. His authority corresponds to his obedience to the higher, symbolic Father, but his desire is frustrated and his masculine position has been given to him. Although he rules the principality abdicated by Manfred, Theodore does not have Manfred's power. The actual phallic power remains in the hands of Alfonso even after he disappears with saint Nicholas, "wrapt from mortal eyes in a blaze of glory" (108).

Otranto, in this way, becomes a land controlled by an absent father who demands obedience and punishes desire. In the end, the ultimate male authorities disappear into the clouds, leaving behind a world placed in their chosen hierarchical order and male characters whose sexual desires have been frustrated. The men who remain in Otranto are without the women they want and, subsequently, symbolically castrated. Jerome has been without his wife, who was taken by corsairs, for years before the narrative begins, and Frederic and Theodore both lose Matilda. While the conclusion reinforces a belief in a structured value system and the regulation of desire, it also makes the masculine roles of these characters unappealing. At the beginning of the novel, Otranto is ruled by Manfred whose character attracts and repels the reader because he appears to have access to unlimited *jouissance*, and the reader's fantasies are engaged by the possibilities. His successor, Theodore, on the other hand, never approaches Manfred's male image, and readers may not see him as a model of successful masculinity. He is a passive character who reacts to the actions of the other characters. Even his combat with Frederic is both a defensive maneuver and a mistake. Because he fails to protect Matilda, he will never have her or the unknown pleasure that she promises as the object of his desire. Although Theodore finally rules Otranto, Manfred remains the strongest male image and symbol for a phallic masculinity in the text.

The marriage at the end should represent for Theodore a symbolic immortality with his union or completion with Isabella, but this immortality is artificial and hollow. He will "forever" (110) lack Matilda whom he tries but fails to marry as she lies dying, and, instead of his soul-mate, "melancholy" (110) possesses his soul. Manfred had sought the forbidden but accessible Isabella as the object of his male fantasy, whereas Theodore hopelessly desires the dead Matilda. Ironically, Theodore gets what Manfred wants, Isabella and the principality, but he can never have what he wants. Legitimacy and order have been restored to Otranto, but the possibility of pleasure, especially forbidden pleasure, has disappeared. With his victory, the Symbolic Other (Alfonso and saint Nicholas) has reinstalled the structured security of a system of rational laws (Theodore and legitimacy) and simultaneously repressed the drives (Manfred and desire), but the world represented at the end of the novel is a world without joy.

Like Richardson's Lovelace, Manfred is vanquished in the plot only to retain his position as the most masculine character in the novel. Just as Belford's happy marriage seems rather benign compared to the unlimited promise of pleasure that Lovelace originally suggests, Theodore's consoling marriage does not compare with the initial unrestrained power that Manfred seemingly wields. By denying his castration and defying the Law which represents a barrier to pleasure and immortality, Walpole's prototypical Gothic villain establishes a pattern of masculine behavior which would be copied by later Gothic writers. Villains like Lewis's Ambrosio and

Radcliffe's Schedoni and Montoni share Manfred's pursuit of the forbidden and form their identities by a mistaken belief in narcissistic completion. While readers may abhor the actions of such villains, they may also share each villain's indulgence in the fantasy of phallic power. Because this fantasy can be attractive, however, the seemingly moral ending of the Gothic novel may be unconvincing and a moral behavior for men is not clearly defined. If readers are attracted to the Gothic novel on the strength of the villain, then the masculine nature of that villain must dominate and, consequently, may be promoted by the novel. This pattern begins with Manfred in Otranto and is copied by every significant Gothic novel which follows. When the Marquis de Sade observed that the Gothic novel was a part of the discourse of revolution,[30] he was referring to the turbulent sexual nature of these novels and the manner in which the villains transgress societal law.

Because of the transgressive nature of its villains, the Gothic novel is regularly described as a "subversive" reaction to the eighteenth century "idea of balance and regularity"[31] and "one tributary of the general revolt against rational structures that would later coalesce into the mighty stream of Romanticism at the end of the century."[32] However, if these novels are "subversive," they are subversive not in the manner in which they would change society but in the way they portray the individual against society, and, in particular, in the power they attribute to a villain who transgresses society's rules. Every individual in Gothic fiction, including the villains, is a potential victim either of some other individual, of an institution like the Church, or of a force outside of nature. Survival in this world is an act of self-interest, and the villains not only survive but thrive in this atmosphere of conflict and terror. Though the Gothic novel, therefore, outwardly promotes social norms and discourages the behavior of

163

the villain, readers may see aspects of this character as important to survival in a changing, more competitive environment which no longer offers the security of an accepted patriarchal structure. In the Gothic, the justice available from this structure is openly questioned, and the larger symbols of patriarchal authority like the Church, the Inquisition, or those who enforce the law are as likely to punish the innocent as the guilty. In Otranto, for example, the innocent fifteen-year-old Conrad is murdered by unseen heavenly powers in order to reestablish the proper lineage for the rulers of the principality. To a certain degree, the villain in every important Gothic novel, like Manfred, outwits this authority and wages a solitary war in pursuit of his own pleasure against the greater powers that would limit that pleasure. If, as David Punter states, "it is historically obvious that the Gothic coincides with a specific stage of the reorganization of English society and economy,"[33] then the Gothic villain's brief triumph suggests an alternative type of male who may have access to a pleasure which is denied to those who are restrained by society and the economy. The subversive nature of the Gothic novel, therefore, relates not to its moral, but to the attraction of its fantasy, the fantasy of power embodied by the villain.

When Horace Walpole wrote The Castle of Otranto, he was looking to reconstruct the past and not revolutionize the future. In his often quoted remarks from the Preface to the second edition, he describes his novel as "an attempt to blend the two kinds of romance, the ancient and the modern" (9). If "he was bored with the insipidity of Richardson and the coarseness of Fielding and Smollett,"[34] he was interested in looking backward to the days before the desire for "only cold reason"[35] and not forward to a world altered by revolutionary principles. While his political sentiments were "Whiggish, libertarian, and antimonarchical,"[36] he was an "Old Whig"[37] who "loved the glamorous past"[38] and who "did not want kings destroyed."[39] He claimed to have written <u>Otranto</u> to "keep his mind off politics,"[40] and the medieval setting as well as the supernatural machinery provided a landscape which distanced him from the troubles of his own time.

What Walpole retains of the modern in his "Gothic story" (15) is the characterization of "mere men and women" (8) as they react to the improbable (and impossible) events of the novel. "Desirous of leaving the powers of fancy at liberty to expatiate through the boundless realms of invention" (7), Walpole creates an alternative world where his villain Manfred wields tyrannical power, but ultimately succumbs to his predestined fate and the hereditary claims of the heroic Theodore. While the creation of this labyrinthine and aberrant world marks a significant departure from Richardson's realism, the male behavior which succeeds and fails in <u>Otranto</u> differs little from that of <u>Clarissa</u>. In much the same way as Lovelace, Manfred opposes the system and maintains power through his own violent presence only to lose everything to a greater, normalizing patriarchal power. As Stephen Bernstein asserts, Gothic novels, like the novels of Richardson, demonstrate that "the power of social stability is stronger than any individual's attempt to transgress it,"[41] but at the same time that the plot of <u>Otranto</u> discourages individual desires and encourages societal conformity and restraint, the novel's interpellative power is derived from the phallic fantasies it evokes. Though obedience to the Law provides characters with a secure position, successful masculinity remains above and outside of the Law. <u>Otranto</u> can be read as socially stabilizing, but the text can also be read as revolutionary and subversive in its portrayal of the individual male against the system. While readers reject Manfred's tyranny, they respond to his power. Perhaps, like the antiquarian who created the first Gothic novel, they long for a mythical time when there was a phallic father who set things right with his Word. Instead, the world is left with a limited sovereign, a passive recipient of male authority, like a son, such as Theodore, and not like a father, an active, generative source.

Notes

[1]Samuel Taylor Coleridge, The Table Talk and Omniana of Samuel Taylor Coleridge (London: Humphrey Milford: Oxford UP, 1917) 297.

[2]See Chapter Two; see also Michael McKeon, "Historicizing Patriarchy: The Emergence of Gender Difference in England, 1660-1760," Eighteenth-Century Studies 28 (1995) 295-322; Thomas Laqueur, Making Sex: Body and Gender from the Greeks to Freud, (Cambridge, MA: Harvard UP, 1990).

[3]George Haggerty, "The Gothic Novel, 1764-1824," The Columbia History of the British Novel, ed. John Richetti (New York: Columbia UP, 1994) 239.

[4]William Patrick Day, In the Circles of Fear and Desire (Chicago: U of Chicago P, 1985) 17.

[5]Day 17.

[6]K. K. Mehrotra, Horace Walpole and the English Novel: A Study of the Influence of "The Castle of Otranto" 1764-1820 (New York: Russell & Russell, 1934, 1970) 25.

[7]Frederick S. Frank, preface, The First Gothics: A Critical Guide to the English Gothic Novel (New York: Garland, 1987) ix.

[8]Day 62-69.

[9]Day 62-69.

[10]Day 17.

[11]Devendra Varma, The Gothic Flame (New York: Russell & Russell, 1966).

[12]Robert Donald Spector, The English Gothic: A Bibliographic Guide to Writers from Horace Walpole to Mary Shelley (Westport, CT: Greenwood, 1984) 83.

[13]Frederick S. Frank, introduction, Gothic Fiction: A Master List of Twentieth Century Criticism and Research (Westport, CT: Meckler, 1988) ix.

[14]Wilmarth Sheldon Lewis, Horace Walpole (New York: Pantheon Books, 1960) 158.

[15]Spector 83.

[16]Lewis 158.

[17]Spector 83.

[18]Spector 91.

[19]Traditional Gothic criticism began with Edith Birkhead's The Tale of Terror: A Study of the Gothic Romance (London: Constable, 1921) and Eino Railo's The Haunted Castle: A Study of the Elements of English Romanticism (London: Routledge, 1927); was revived by Monteque Summers' The Gothic Quest (New York: Russell & Russell, 1964) and Varma's The Gothic Flame; and continued with David Punter's The Literature of Terror: A History of Gothic Fictions from 1765 to the Present Day (London: Longman, 1980). Varma, in particular, describes the significance of Walpole's novel by showing how his Gothic machinery established a set of fictional elements which later writers copied.

[20]Varma sees Manfred as a direct foreshadowing of the Byronic hero, 60; Peter Thorslev, however, sees the Gothic villain as only one antecedent of what he views as Byron's more complex creation in The Byronic Hero: Types and Prototypes,, Minneapolis: U of Minn P, 1962. It is also, perhaps, significant to note that Byron admired Walpole's novel and borrowed the name of Otranto's villain for the hero and the title of his Faustian poetic drama, Manfred.

[21]Frank, preface, The First Gothics, ix.

[22]Betsy Perteit Harfst, Horace Walpole and the Unconscious: an Experiment in Freudian Analysis (New York: Arno Press, 1980); Martin Kallich, Horace Walpole (New York: Twayne, 1971) 102-103.

[23]Kallich 95.

[24]Lewis 20.

[25]Lewis 24.

[26]Horace Walpole, The Yale Edition of Horace Walpole's Correspondence, vol. 10, ed. W. S. Lewis (London: Humphrey Milford: Oxford UP, 1941) 192.

[27]Lars E. Troide, introduction, Horace Walpole's Miscellany 1786-1795 (New Haven: Yale UP, 1978) xxviii.

[28]Mark Bracher, Lacan, Discourse, and Social Change: A Psychoanalytic Cultural Criticism (Ithaca: Cornell UP, 1993) 49.

[29]Bracher 116.

[30]De Sade thought that "the appearance of [The Monk] was truly a literary event. It answered the need for strong emotions following great upheavals, flattered sensualism with its voluptuous pictures and irreligion by the boldness with which it treated sacred things." qtd in Varma, 150-151.

[31]Spector 6

[32]Frank, preface, xix.

[33]David Punter, "Narrative and Psychology in Gothic Fiction," Gothic Fictions: Prohibition/Transgression, ed. Kenneth W. Graham (New York: AMS, 1989) 10.

[34]Lewis 161.

[35]qtd. in Lewis 161.

[36]Kallich 34.

[37]Kallich 33.

[38]Kallich 27.

[39]Kallich 63.

[40]Lewis 161.

[41]Stephen Bernstein, "Form and Ideology in the Gothic Novel," Essays in Literature 18 (1991) 153.

CHAPTER VI

MATTHEW LEWIS AND THE MASCULINE OTHER

Wide as I've roam'd the world around,

Roam where I would, I ever found,

The worst of Women still possest

More virtues than of Men the best.

from "Landing" by M. G. Lewis[1]

While Horace Walpole gave his villain a straightforward goal, the retention of sovereignty, and a generally unambiguous character, later Gothic writers would develop the Gothic hero-villain by attempting to disclose more of his motivations. An increased interest in the emotional workings of characters, exemplified by the cult of sensibility,[2] and a fascination with the sublime terror described by Edmund Burke in <u>A Philosophical Enquiry into the Origin of Our Ideas of the Sublime and the Beautiful</u> was reflected both in the subtle terrors of Ann Radcliffe's dark but scenic landscapes and in the growing "crescendo of emotion"[3] produced by the novels of Matthew Lewis and Charles Maturin. What results are male characters who resemble Manfred in their disregard for societal laws, but who desire a narcissistic gratification which, unlike Manfred, has no basis in the traditional hierarchical structure. A character like Lewis's Ambrosio, for example, who is driven to sell his soul for the desires of the flesh, resembles Richardson's Lovelace, a competitive male whose own actions define him, more than Walpole's Manfred, who clings to an established, albeit illegitimate, patriarchal power. In contrast to Manfred, who loses his principality because he is not the rightful heir, Ambrosio loses his authority and his life because he is unable to check his sexual desires and is willing to do anything, including the selling of his soul, to remain alive. In Lewis's hands, the Gothic villain is a man whose male sexual desires turn him into a monster, and his atrocities and ultimate destruction demonstrate the disastrous consequences of male desire.

Although Ambrosio's primary goal in The Monk is the sexual conquest of Antonia, he is not, like Lovelace, a libertine who enjoys a game of pursuing females and is frustrated by a woman who resists him. Instead, Ambrosio is driven solely by physical lust to rape the object of his desire, and his confrontation with authority occurs because of his inability to reconcile the demands of society (which insists that he be chaste) and his interest in sexual pleasure. Unlike Lovelace, therefore, who uses the discourse of the libertine to hide the fantasy of phallic completion and immortality, Ambrosio's discourse of desire reveals a fantasy of pleasure associated with the female body and located outside of society's rules for sexual behavior. Furthermore, while Richardson juxtaposed Lovelace's discourse against the moral discourse of Clarissa, Lewis provides only a weak counter-discourse which steers the other male characters, who have potentially similar desires to Ambrosio, into marriages rather than criminal behavior. For the majority of Lewis's characters, possession of the Other as a means of one's *jouissance* (active anaclitic desire) remains of primary importance, and love (active narcissistic desire) has a minimal significance.[4] Ultimately, The Monk is not about good and evil identities, but about the body, the hypocritical demands which society places upon the sexuality of the individual, and, paradoxically, the evil which is inherent in sexual desire, a desire which males, in particular, find difficult to resist.

Unlike Radcliffe's earlier The Mysteries of Udolpho, which pitted its unprotected heroine Emily against a series of external threats, The Monk's conflict occurs internally as each character's individual sexuality struggles with the limitations of the sexual roles imposed by society and authority. In the words of Kenneth Graham, "The Monk questions restriction through attacks on enforced repressions as a series of authority figures, including church and family, deny to children outlets for their passions."[5] In addition, as David Punter has pointed out, Lewis's novel has the effect of showing the reader "unwholesome and repressed aspects of his own psyche,"[6] and this emphasis on the inner horrors rather than those horrors imposed from outside powers "puts [the reader] in touch," according to Peter Brooks, "not with Godhead, but with the unconscious."[7] Although there are supernatural forces in The Monk, the true "daemons represent not a wholly other, but a complex of interdicted erotic desires within us."[8] In Lewis's text, therefore, sexual desires become demons, but they do so because of the unnatural bondage established by the Catholic Church and by an older generation which demands submission to its unjust authority.

This resistance to the demands of authority presented by Lewis's characters seems to have arisen more from the circumstances of the nineteen-year-old author's life than from any desire to create a subversive text (or one which was a part of the discourse of revolution, as The Monk was labeled by the Marquis de Sade).[9] When he wrote his first and only novel, the young Lewis was bored with his position as attaché to the British embassy in The Hague and interested more in earning money from writing than in creating any kind of philosophical or political stir. The Monk was composed quickly, "in the space of ten weeks,"[10] according to its author in a letter to his mother, but previous letters indicate that Lewis had been writing "most furiously"[11] for a few years in hopes of producing a play, a poem, or a novel which would earn him the fame and monetary independence he sought so that he could financially help his mother, who had separated from his father when Lewis was six. Inspired by Radcliffe's Udolpho, which he described as "one of the most interesting books that has ever been published,"[12] Lewis combined European eroticism, French anti-clericalism, and German supernaturalism in a unique manner that surprised and pleased his English readership. Using two plots, both of which are a series of episodes interspersed with a series of poems, Lewis used all that he had found most fascinating in the stories he had heard, seen on stage, or read, and then, setting his young imagination free, he told a story of his own.

Primarily, The Monk is the story of Ambrosio, an abbot of the Capuchins and a man of thirty who until the time of the novel has been shielded from society and its vices by the walls of an abbey. The main narrative shows Ambrosio's fall from his arrogantly held position of esteem and power, but the strength of Lewis's text is found in his presentation of individual scenes. By focusing the story on the villain rather than on his victims, unlike Walpole and Radcliffe, Lewis not only gives a psychologically believable portrait of a vain man's seduction into evil but also shows how attractive temptation can be. Like Richardson's Lovelace, Ambrosio defines himself apart from society's laws and seeks those pleasures denied to the law-abiding, and, although he becomes undeniably evil, Ambrosio initially shares with Lovelace the potential for a *jouissance* and a masculine authority that the other male characters do not possess. However, Ambrosio does not control his world like Lovelace, but instead falls victim to its corrupting influence. While Lovelace is the master manipulator in Clarissa, Ambrosio is manipulated, first, by Matilda, and later, by his own desires.

Masculinity in <u>The Monk</u> is not revealed as a contest between male types, but is shown as an interior battle with sexual desire. By introducing Ambrosio as a man who has never experienced temptation, Lewis is able to show the deleterious progress of a man who follows his sexual impulses. Lewis maintains his reader's interest through his ability to create repeated scenes of restrained and unleashed desire, a device which occurs most effectively in Ambrosio's relationship with Matilda, who initiates the monk first into carnality and then into necromancy before ultimately encouraging him to sign his soul away to Lucifer. Eventually, however, when Ambrosio sates himself with Matilda's flesh and then pursues the naïve and virginal Antonia for the pleasure found in a new form of depravity, Lewis establishes a pattern of sexual desire, sexual conquest, and revulsion toward the sexual object. Nevertheless, Lewis does not present Ambrosio as a reluctant victim of desire, but as a man unable to control himself who is tempted by a woman who encourages his desires. All men in the text are understood to be seeking sexual pleasure; the only checks on their desires come from those women who exhibit virtuous conduct.

The episodic structure of the text duplicates this pleasure-seeking pattern by stimulating interest, satisfying curiosity, and leading the reader to the next episode, which promises to be even more provocative than the last. Critics have often sought out sources for Lewis's scenes, and he no doubt borrowed considerably from folk tales, myths, and other authors; however, his willingness to go to extremes to affect his readers has few, if any, precedents. Ambrosio gazes at the naked Antonia in an enchanted mirror; he uses a magic myrtle to gain access to her bedchamber, where he is thwarted by her mother Elvira, whom he kills; and finally he drugs Antonia so that she appears dead and so that he may later rape her amid the corpses in the vault where she has been interred. When he is discovered there, he kills her. Having done all of this, Ambrosio learns from Lucifer that Elvira was his mother and Antonia was his sister. As if the crimes themselves were not enough, Lewis gives his readers some *ex post facto* matricide and incest. Scheduled to be punished for these crimes by the Inquisition, Ambrosio gives his soul to Lucifer, who promptly pierces Ambrosia's skull with his talons, carries him into the sky, and drops him down a rocky precipice to die by a river. Unable to move to satisfy a burning thirst, Ambrosio dies slowly, tormented by scavenging birds and insects, over a period of six days.

The fantasy ($ \$ <> \underline{a} $) which the plot promotes, therefore, follows Ambrosio's search for physical pleasure through his sexual adventures, which promise an unknown and forbidden *jouissance* ($\underline{a}$), to his symbolic castration at the hands of an even more powerful male. This fantasy continually presents the Woman as the object for masculine desire (in the register of the Real), the female body as a sexual object (in the Imaginary register), and identifies men and women by societally-sanctioned and naturally oppositional roles (the Symbolic register), associations which, according to Mark Bracher, are features of pornography. In addition, Lewis's text also resembles pornography in its focus on sexual difference and on an innate need for the sexes to have each other.[13] Rather than privileging the penis as phallus, however, as pornography does, Lewis's text repeatedly shows the inability of the penis to provide satisfaction for either the male or the female. In The Monk, phallic power, or the power often associated with sexual conquest and male domination, is a disruptive and disturbing force. Where Richardson and Walpole create good and evil uses for male power, all male power in The Monk has horrific results. The novel is sexual because of its continued interest in male/female difference and desire, but it is perverse because it does not resolve this difference by placing the power which Ambrosio forfeits into the hands of another, morally acceptable male (like Richardson's Belford or Walpole's Theodore). Instead, Lucifer triumphs, and the self-interested actions of all the characters, especially the male characters, support a conclusion that the Gothic world which Lewis creates cannot sustain virtue.

The morality of Lewis's characters changes from one page to the next, so that not only does Ambrosio fall from purity to depravity, but the other characters also demonstrate inconsistent virtue. Agnes and Raymond, the heroine and hero of a second story line which intersects the text, betray family and church and have a child out of wedlock. Lorenzo, Agnes's brother, has his friend Don Christoval feign interest in Antonia's matronly aunt Leonella so Lorenzo can spend time alone with Antonia. None of the characters appears above subterfuge, and all are ready victims for their passions. Although Ambrosio's transgression is to be carried away by his desires, all of the characters lose restraint when given an opportunity for a sexual encounter. The men, particularly Lorenzo and Raymond, use all means possible to gain the objects of their desire, and the women, Agnes, Leonella, and Agnes's aunt, Donna Rodolpha, need only a word of encouragement "to yield," as Donna Rodolpha says to Raymond, "to the violence of . . . passion."[14] In contrast to these characters, Ambrosio's sin becomes a matter of a difference in degree and not kind, and his use of necromancy and violence seems only an extension of the opportunity offered to him that the others do not have. After all, his motive, the fulfillment of desire, does not separate him from the other characters.

Impelled by sexual desire, the characters who safely direct their energies toward marriage, a course Lorenzo, Raymond, and Agnes follow, find happiness and security at the end of the novel, although

175

that happiness is tempered by their mortality which makes them the "prey of grief, and sport of disappointment" (400). Those who ignore the sexual boundaries of their marriage like Donna Rodolpha and those who do not direct their passions toward an intended marriage like Ambrosio and Matilda are eventually and eternally punished for this lack of restraint. On the other hand, however, avoidance or refusal to admit desire also leads to disastrous results. After all, Ambrosio's inability to cope with his newly awakened sexuality stems in part from his seclusion in the cloister:

> For a time spare diet, frequent watching, and severe penance cooled and repressed the natural warmth of his constitution: but no sooner did opportunity present itself, no sooner did he catch a glimpse of joys to which he was still a stranger, than religion's barriers were too feeble to resist the overwhelming torrent of his desires. (239-240)

Ambrosio's education and life with the Capuchins are against his "nature" (239), but there is little evidence, if any, in the text of anyone whose nature agrees with the checks on passion imposed by celibacy. On the contrary, the action of the text takes the characters away from the convent, the locus of unnatural confinement, and toward marriage, where desires are satisfactorily fulfilled, or death where unrestrained desires inevitably end. Virginia and Agnes escape the convent and marry Lorenzo and Raymond; Ambrosio, of course, does not escape.

Lewis establishes the unnatural and hypocritical relationship between seemingly chaste authority and sexuality on the first page of the novel, beginning with a reference to Measure for Measure's sanctimonious Lord Angelo, whose "appetite is more to bread than stone" (35). Though The Monk may be read as showing this hypocrisy as part of the evils of Catholicism, the more prominent deceit in the novel occurs in the minds of the characters who, like Lord Angelo, outwardly profess religious principles while being inwardly driven by unrighteous motives. The Capuchin church in the first scene is not a site of "true devotion" (35), but a place where people gather out of vanity and idleness, and the true interest of these people is not for religion but for each other as "one half of Madrid was brought thither by expecting to meet the other half" (35). In other words, the Church fails to fulfill its function because people are corrupt, but the Church remains a social construction which serves to bring people into contact with each other. As the remainder of The Monk will show, human interaction invariably fosters sexual interest, so the Church functions to create an atmosphere of desire by bringing bodies into social contact and then demanding unrealistic restraints.

On this site of sexual tension (at the church), Lewis quickly maps out the difference between his male and female characters. Both willingly enter the sexual arena because each desires the other; however, their roles differ once they arrive. "The women came to show themselves, the men to see the women" (35). The men gaze; the women are objects of the gaze. This traditional position of the two genders[15] is complicated, however, by the nature of female participation in the event. First of all, the women are active participants: they desire to be seen. Secondly, they control the location of the encounter: the men are at the church because of the women. If the women are elsewhere, the men would apparently have followed. In this way, women have a power that men do not, and although men in this scenario control the sexual exchange by choosing the objects they will gaze upon, women initiate this exchange by making themselves available. Though the limitations of this power might seem stereotypical, developments later in the text show that this initial female control opens the door to unbridled (un-brided) female power. Most of the female characters have the potential to act on their desires and to use their sexuality to enflame and control men. Those women who are to be viewed as morally good, like Antonia and Agnes, resist taking this action.

Unlike females, male characters in <u>The Monk</u> are constants. Put into contact with a sexually desirable woman, each acts to possess her physically. Ambrosio's "see flesh, have flesh" pattern, because of his long seclusion, emphasizes this male characteristic, but readers are assumed to accept the unrelenting and unvaried nature of the male sex drive. When Raymond rejects the advances of Donna Rodolpha, he proves his love for Agnes and his honor for the baron, but even this self-control of male desire is mitigated because Rodolpha is "about forty" (146) and only "possessed some remains" (147) of her charms. Men in <u>The Monk</u> are shown as natural sexual instigators, and their refusal of sex apparently requires an explanation. Women, on the other hand, also have desires, but they must show restraint if there is to be any sexual order. Like the harlots who abet Lovelace in <u>Clarissa</u>, Lewis's female characters outdo his male characters in depravity when they yield to their sexual desires.

In the text, unleashed female sexuality threatens masculinity and male power by denying male choice. Implied in Raymond's rejection of Rodolpha is the acknowledgment that if she were unmarried, younger, or her charms greater, Raymond's resistance would create questions about his masculinity. In other words, if a woman is able to choose her sexual partners, the man or the type of masculinity chosen would be dependent on feminine prerogative. In Raymond's case, he maintains his masculinity because the woman he refuses is not a young beauty, and he does not need to deny himself a seemingly great physical pleasure. Lewis's emphasis on Rodolpha's diminished physical attractiveness underscores his repeated focus on desire instead of love as the motivation for sexual relationships.

He also shows how a woman who acts on her desires and makes sexual advances creates a dilemma for the masculine norm: a man can refuse and deny his male sexual imperative or accept and cede control to the female. Because these choices place the woman in power, traditional masculinity requires female desires to be held in check, and Lewis tenuously maintains male authority in the text by showing disastrous results for those women who go too far.

In The Monk, while both male and female characters are motivated by sexual desire, the consequences of acting on those desires are different for the two genders. Except for Ambrosio, the male characters are excused for their desires. When Lorenzo is told about his sister Agnes's seduction by Raymond, for example, he forgives his friend (after a momentary reaction of anger) with the justification: "The temptation was too great to be resisted" (198). The female characters are not exonerated in the same way: Agnes suffers physical torment and has her baby die in her arms, Leonella is viewed as comically "affected" and "ridiculous" (246), Marguerite is suffered to live as the wife of a bandit whom she does not love, Beatrice (the Bleeding Nun) is stabbed to death, and Donna Rodolpha appears vulgar, predatory, and spiteful and dies when she breaks "a blood-vessel" (199). While Lewis's text posits the presence of female sexual passion, it discourages any actions resulting from that passion by establishing a gender-based system of punishment which results in a rather conventional rendering of the sexual double standard.

All women, however, are not punished equally in the text because all do not act equally. In order to separate the heroines (Antonia, Agnes, Marguerite) from the female predators (Matilda, Donna Rodolpha, Beatrice), Lewis provided the villainesses with an element of cruelty which the heroines do not have. These women either kill or attempt to kill those who prevent them from getting what they want. In contrast, the only male characters to show this type of sadistic behavior are the banditti and Ambrosio. In both cases, however, circumstances exist which make the male violence more passive and less premeditated than the female. The banditti attack only those who venture into their forest, and they kill for money and not power. Ambrosio murders Elvira and Antonia because he panics and fears they will expose him. In contrast, the evil women act wantonly, premeditating the malicious actions which will bring them possession of a man's soul, body, or barony. All three villainesses do more than desire men; they assume a masculine role by adopting cruel methods and a desire for power traditionally associated with men. In spite of the ultimate deaths of Beatrice and Rodolpha and the demonization of Matilda, these women demonstrate a female power which threatens to surpass male authority.

Simultaneously desirable and desiring, Matilda, Beatrice, and Rodolpha display both male and female characteristics and subsequently dominate those around them. When that which is desired, the female body, also possesses desires for sexual and political dominion, then the woman has a potential power that the man does not. Acting with "the incontinence of a prostitute" (182), the fallen nun Beatrice seduces both a baron and his brother and like the later baroness, Donna Rodolpha, actually controls the castle of Lindenberg. Just as Rodolpha "governed her husband with despotic sway" (156), Beatrice uses her sexual powers to reign over the previous baron, but, in fear of her, her accomplice to the baron's murder, his brother Otto, kills her. Without violence, men seem powerless against desirable women who want to usurp male control. In The Monk, once female desire is recognized, only the possibility of pregnancy, which happens to Agnes, and the loss of reputation, which Elvira tries to shield Antonia against, can keep women from exercising this power. Without restraint, female desire threatens to create anarchy by removing barriers which structure gender divisions and social controls on the deployment of sexuality.

Nowhere is this clearer than in the character of Matilda. Introduced in the text as the novice monk Rosario, Matilda behaves "with sweetness" (66), "reserve" (66), and "docility" (67) as a male, but becomes increasingly aggressive once her actual sex and her love for Ambrosio are "unveiled" (80). In her role as a woman in love, Matilda cannot avoid the complexities of seduction. Though she vows that she would never "endeavor to seduce" (85) Ambrosio, she repeatedly asserts her love and refuses to quit the monastery. When Ambrosio threatens to force her away, she draws a dagger and places the point against her "half exposed" left breast, a "beauteous orb" of "dazzling whiteness." This sight makes Ambrosio's "blood boil," and evokes his verbal reaction: "Stay then, enchantress!" (87). Though Matilda has acted only upon herself, she has acted to inflame Ambrosio's desires. Once she voices her desire for Ambrosio and reveals her female body, he is no longer in control. Earlier, Ambrosio had been the teacher, "instructing [Rosario] in various sciences" (67), but now Matilda directs the action. She is a "seducing object" (98), an oxymoron that describes her simultaneously active and passive nature, and she also becomes superior to "the superior" (67), simply by expressing her desire and revealing her bosom.

Because Matilda pursues Ambrosio, the object of her desire, while being herself an erotically appealing object (for male desire), nothing can prevent her from getting what she wants. After Ambrosio breaks his vow of celibacy with her, she becomes the teacher, putting "every invention of lust in practice, every refinement in the art of pleasure, which might heighten the bliss of her possession, and render her lover's transports still more exquisite" (227). Matilda is now the "fair wanton" and the "syren" (227) who "possesses" Ambrosio, and his future acts of depravity will happen with her encouragement and aid. With her new authority, her personality changes and she steps out of her gender role. "Now she assumed a sort of courage and manliness in her manners and discourse" and "spoke no longer to insinuate, but command" (233). Furthermore, while Matilda expresses her female desire when she declares "the woman reigns in my bosom, and I am become a prey to the wildest of passions" (233), her efforts to satisfy those desires change her from a "fond," "gentle," and "submissive" male (Rosario) to an "unfeminine" (234) and commanding female. Apparently, the assumption of a male persona does not alter her feminine position, but her aroused desire does. When Lewis essentially unsexes her character by disclosing at the end that she was a demon all along, he negates the power Matilda acquires through the unrestrained use of her sexuality. Before this disclosure, her final scene demonstrates the boundlessness of her sexual desires and of her mastery of her circumstances:

> I will enjoy unrestrained the gratification of my senses; every passion shall be indulged even to satiety; then will I bid my servants invent new pleasures, to revive and stimulate my glutted appetites! (233)

Adopting a desire for sexual gratification traditionally viewed as male and unchecked by moral limitations, Matilda is a "dangerous woman" (226), who epitomizes the evil and powerful potential of unrestrained female sexuality. Only Lewis's attempt to undo her role as woman can undermine this conclusion.

Before she is demonized, Matilda clearly represents the most masculine female in the text, not only due to her appearance as both man and woman, but also because she is the first in the text to "penetrate" (234) the subterranean vaults between the abbey and convent, and she also engineers Ambrosio's abduction, rape, and murder of Antonia. By instruction and example, she shows Ambrosio how to be a man by introducing him to the pleasures of sex and the abuses of power. At the other extreme, Antonia represents the most feminine female, never acting on her own in the novel and remaining so naïve and without desire that she cannot understand the concept of romantic love and has a "virgin's terror" (259) when she considers what her husband's desires will be. All the other female characters, with the exception of Elvira, whose role as mother seems to preclude sexuality, occupy positions more active or desiring than Antonia but less than Matilda. Within this spectrum of possible female sexualities, a pattern emerges that shows women hopelessly trapped in a world which preys upon them if they know too little, but punishes them if they have any desire whatsoever. Sexual desire, however, is inherent in all the women, a fact acknowledged by Elvira when she expurgates Antonia's bible because "many of the narratives can only tend to excite ideas the worst calculated for a female breast" (258). In The Monk, the test for female virtue is not an absence of desire, but a tempering of desire combined with a knowledge of passion's consequences which keeps the female from utilizing her seductive power and encroaching on masculine authority.

Men in the novel, however, abuse masculine authority in their own way. The marquis de la Cisternas disinherits his son Gonzalvo for marrying Elvira and subsequently puts in motion the tragic events of the novel by placing the infant Ambrosio in a cloister. Don Gaston de Medici unfairly supports his sister Rodolpha's proposal to confine Agnes in a convent. "The abbot, a very monk," brainwashes the young Ambrosio by using "all his endeavours to persuade the boy that happiness existed not without the walls of a convent" (238). Because of these abuses of patriarchal power, the younger generation suffers and must work to correct the injustices caused by their predecessors. At the end of the novel, the older generation is dead and Lorenzo and Raymond use their inherited wealth and power to put things right by marrying and joining their two families. Nevertheless, Ambrosio endures tortures and dies for the sins he commits as a result of the circumstances he is born into and the training he has received.

At the beginning of The Monk, Ambrosio appears as a blank slate upon which the Capuchins have etched their beliefs. Without wealth and without knowledge of his parents, Ambrosio receives from the monks an identity which defines him as a "present . . . from the virgin" (44) and which initially marks him as a Christ-like figure. This pious veneer, however, has been artificially established by total seclusion from the world, and when the story begins three months after Ambrosio's introduction into society, "the brilliance of his virtue" is "thrown into the way of temptation" (48) for the first time. Nevertheless, instead of showing Ambrosio's subsequent seduction and descent into depravity as the failure of his virtue, Lewis describes Ambrosio's inner conflict as a battle between his "education and nature" (239), which his nature wins. Driven by "the cravings of brutal appetite" and a "constitution" which makes "a woman necessary to him" (237), Ambrosio does not hesitate long when given the opportunity to break his vows. He cannot control his passions, and his lack of worldly experience provides him with little defense against Matilda's suggestions and seductive supplications.

Like all the major male characters, Ambrosio is in "the full vigour of manhood" (109), but his "unnatural" (227) upbringing creates conditions which heighten his susceptibility to sensual stimulation.[16] This misfeasance of his educators provides a Rousseauvian explanation for Ambrosio's defenseless naïveté; however, his first problem is

184

that he is a man and has a man's desires. On one level, readers can understand and even share these desires. Ambrosio's interest in Matilda's exposed breast and his curiosity to view the undressing Antonia in Matilda's magic mirror is reproduced in the reader's fascination with these erotic scenes. In voyeuristic fashion, Ambrosio and the reader share the complex position of empowered observers, possessing and obtaining pleasure from what they see in fantasy, but remaining at a safe distance from the action.[17] While readers later abandon any sympathies they may have for Ambrosio when he begins to act violently, they continue to duplicate his desire for more and greater sensational pleasures. In addition, through his unabated attempt to achieve sexual satisfaction, the character of Ambrosio provides The Monk with a masculine presence which provides coherence for this episodic text.

Although when he initially appears Ambrosio has the "power, authority, and control"[18] that identify him as a representative of phallic sovereignty, this power is suspect. Immediately, Leonella questions his heritage, assuming that he must be the son of a noble, and Lorenzo, Antonia's legitimate suitor and a nobleman, suggests that Ambrosio has not accomplished anything until he shows that he can resist worldly temptation. Despite all of his authority, Ambrosio lacks a masculine identity because his education has neutered him, leaving him ignorant of "the difference of man and woman" (44), and he has no patriarchal link to the aristocratic world of Lorenzo and Raymond. His "surname" of "The Man of Holiness" when he begins the novel is not inherited from a benevolent father-image, but the result of years of study, an acquisition of profound knowledge, and a persuasive and enchanting rhetorical ability. He is a self-made man, but the man he has created neither fulfills the prerequisites of hierarchical maleness nor the essential characteristics of biological manhood. As Lorenzo points out, Ambrosio's initial image of male completeness is a false one. By the end of the text, Ambrosio acquires his hereditary identity and "proves" his maleness by sexual relations with women, and, in doing so, he sheds his artificial image as "a saint" while establishing his masculinity through his actions; nevertheless, all this identity brings him is his own destruction.

Just as Richardson's Lovelace carves out his own masculine identity in defiance of hierarchical authority, Ambrosio ignores that authority to create his "self" through the pursuit of his own desires. Ambrosio also shares Lovelace's mistaken belief that possession of a specific female body, either that of Antonia or Clarissa, somehow has a meaning beyond the physical circumstances of the sex act. Because, as I have shown in Chapter Four, Lovelace seeks a love from an Other which will recognize and esteem him, he loses everything when Clarissa escapes him and eventually goes to her father's house in heaven; however, Ambrosio has no need to be loved. The Monk is solely about anaclitic desire (the desire to possess and be possessed by the other) and its characters consistently recognize this desire in place of love. If Ambrosio and Antonia had derived pleasure from their sexual union, this privileging of penis as phallus would have, as I suggested earlier, given the novel the features of pornography, but Lewis repeatedly shows the failure of the penis to provide the desired *jouissance*. Instead, men are ineffective sexually compared to the women who can control them by seduction and refusal. Rather than rejecting female sexuality, as Jacqueline Howard suggests,[19] Lewis privileges the female with the capacity to control sexual relations and shows how sexual desire destroys what is virtuous in women. In other words, Lewis shows the female as not only the Madonna but also the whore, and his male characters, while desiring both, find themselves unable to please either.

Ambrosio's masculinity, in outline, develops from an initial feminine-like state as an object for public view to passive voyeur to aggressive seducer to cruel rapist, but Lewis's own ambiguity toward his characters makes Ambrosio's sexuality more complex and problematic. Haggerty, Eve Kosofsky Sedgwick and Linda Bayer-Berenbaum have speculated that Lewis's homosexual desires colored the text,[20] and there is evidence in the text of the attraction of young men like Rosario and Theodore, Raymond's servant. Nevertheless, the nature and extent of Lewis's sexual activities and interests remain historically unclear[21] and attempting to locate textual evidence to label him as a homosexual writer indeed covers up the larger, more obvious problem of a masculinity uncomfortable with itself. Ambrosio begins The Monk in harmony with both the father, the church and papal authority, and the mother, the "Madona" (sic), before whose picture he kneels and prays. By the end, however, he aligns himself with a new father, Lucifer, and he destroys the Madona's picture, sates himself on Matilda, whose likeness the picture bears, and kills his biological mother.

Ambrosio's sexual desire for the mother creates Oedipal questions regarding his relationship to the father, but Ambrosio's biological father is dead and the restrictions which would coincide with the father's presence are not present (apparently not even in the teachings of the church). Ambrosio's actions show disregard of the Law of the Father that dictates kinship relations and societal conduct, and his general lack of guilt or remorse demonstrates that he has formed his subjective identity with little regard for the father's word. Of course, the father's word as it has been communicated from the church and aristocracy is hypocritical and itself perverse, so Ambrosio's conduct suggests a masculinity formed by a son whose Oedipal conflict is not resolved "normally" because the father is symbolically ineffectual. On one hand, therefore, Ambrosio represents a masculinity unfettered by Oedipal restraints; on the other hand, he suffers because he has no authority figure who could have provided him with an identity that would have balanced his sexual drives with the rules of society. At the same time Ambrosio possesses a freedom from sexual restraint and a possibility of pleasure that readers may find attractive, he also reflects the conflict between the drives and societal restrictions to which readers might relate. Without a credible male authority, those restrictions appear sanctimonious and arbitrary. The dominance of desire in Lewis's Gothic world demonstrates the failure and futility of these rules.

The only time Lewis places an emphasis on love is in Ambrosio's relationship to the Madona's, or the mother's, picture, but even this love is destroyed by this omnipresent desire. In this text, the role of the mother is ambiguous because she represents the object of desire both ideally (narcissistic desire) and sexually (anaclitic desire). At first, the image of the Madona symbolizes not only motherhood in its perfection but also Ambrosio's link with immortality. She has "beauty," "sweetness," and "majesty" in an "ideal" sense that transcends "the failings of mortality" (65). In the physical world, however, the Madona is embodied by Matilda, who can provide sexual pleasure but who also leads Ambrosio to mortal suffering and the abandonment of his soul. The Madona is thus the "Virgin" (63) whom Ambrosio will call "the prostitute" (244) when her image is associated with the lascivious Matilda.

In a similar way, Elvira, the vigilant and devoted mother, and Antonia, the naïve and pious female mirror of the earlier, untainted Ambrosio, combine to form a female otherness with whom the monk longs to connect; however, the mother half of this female dyad does not represent a Platonic ideal, but a moral one. She recites the moral lessons in the text and is the sole barrier to unrestricted passion. Until he kills Elvira, Ambrosio is thwarted in his attempts to satisfy his sexual desires with the body of Antonia, and it is Elvira's resistance and not Antonia's which keeps Ambrosio from "the gratification of his lust" (295). However, this resistance only strengthens his resolve and increases his desire. The female obstruction presented by the combination of Elvira and Antonia is removed when Ambrosio completes a planned rape of the drugged daughter with the unplanned murder of the mother. When the action is completed, both are side by side on the same bed, and Ambrosio has taken the pillow from under Antonia's head to smother Elvira. Instead of being on top of the daughter, he ends the scene on top of the mother, symbolically attacking her womb by "pressing his knee upon her stomach with all his strength" (297). Like the destruction of the Madona's image, Elvira's death is caused by Ambrosio's attempt to physically possess her sexual counterpart. Consequently, the mother is simultaneously the source of and the barrier to sexual pleasure, so the ultimate sexual embrace requires her complicity and her resistance, and she must be possessed and destroyed.

Ambrosio's yearning for the mother's image and his subsequent destruction of that image discloses a sexuality driven by a desire for a narcissistic reunification with the mother but repelled by what that sexual union means. On the one hand, Ambrosio can hope to find sexual satisfaction only in those images of his other self: the novice Rosario, the Madona-like Matilda, and his artless sister Antonia; on the other hand, physical possession of this other self does not satisfy his desire and changes the object of love into something which fills him with "aversion and rage"(368). In this way, his attempt to fulfill himself through the satisfaction of male sexual desire fails even before he suffers the deadly consequences of his actions. He mistakenly believes that penetration of his "other" will provide him with some undefined pleasure. Instead, after he succeeds in his design, he shudders "at himself" (368), and curses Matilda and Antonia. The physical enjoyment centered on the penis leads to a feeling of revulsion toward the woman and toward male desire. The penis becomes that which turns the Madona into the whore and destroys any hope of the male's reunification with the ideal Virgin Mother. Ambrosio's identity as a male ultimately prohibits his happiness and leads to his damnation.

At the end of <u>The Monk</u> when Ambrosio rapes Antonia, his rape, like Lovelace's rape of Clarissa, demonstrates his failure to seduce her in spite of his "uncommonly handsome" (45) appearance, celebrated reputation, and persistent entreaties. Antonia triumphs because she refuses to "yield to [her] passions" (367), as Ambrosio instructs her, and consequently rejects the penis as a site of power and an object of desire. Just as Matilda's appropriation of male desire provided her with a power beyond that of men, Antonia's refusal to acknowledge the power of Ambrosio's sexuality disables him. Although he tries to implicate her in the act, he recognizes that, unlike his earlier sexual encounters with Matilda, his rape of Antonia does not reinforce a masculinity built upon the power of male desire. On the contrary, after the rape Ambrosio no longer voices the desires which through-out the text have defined his character: "Of the desires which had urged him to the crime, no trace was left in his bosom" (370). At this point, Ambrosio does not possess the male sexual drive which pro-vided him with a masculine identity beyond his authoritative position. When he attempts to flee persecution for his crimes but is caught and exposed, he forfeits even that position. His symbolic castration is completed as he awaits his pending execution in the dungeon, "ashamed of himself" (411) and without courage.

Male desire has turned the saintly Ambrosio into a self-described "monster" (271), and, in the end, he longs to be reunited with the demonic Matilda instead of the heavenly Madona and signs his soul away to Lucifer. While Antonia has a peaceful death because she knows that she is going to be with her mother, Ambrosio gives himself to his new father and prepares to suffer the horrors of eternal damnation. Heaven, as the home of Elvira and Antonia, represents a place for those who reject male desire, and, by extension, a place that men are incapable of attaining. Ultimately, The Monk is about male failure and the "monstrous" (409) nature of men. Beneath this tale of fluctuating passion and remorse, a vision exists of a hideous and oppressive masculinity which annihilates women and fails to bring pleasure to men.

Lewis claimed that his novel conveyed a moral message,[22] and critic R. D. Hume agrees that The Monk supports a moral norm,[23] but the pleasure of the text for the reader does not occur in its normative ending in the marriage of stock characters and the punishment of the villain. Instead, readers enjoy the book's disjunctive qualities and are drawn to its recurring promise to supply details of a pleasure outside of the law. From the fragmented images of decomposition and mutilation to the descriptions of obscure passageways and dark chambers, the reader's imagination is challenged to make sense of a literary world where the only constant is a sexual desire which pits the individual against an older, disingenuous authority. The Monk's subversive power comes from its ability to involve the reader in an identification process that requires a choice between individual desire and authoritative restraint. Once the reader engages in the fantasy of unlimited sexual pleasure that Matilda offers to Ambrosio, he or she takes Lucifer's side and, in spite of the revolting images and actions which follow, enjoys voyeuristically all the frustrations and pleasures of Ambrosio.

Ambrosio and Matilda emerge from the novel as individuals whose identity and circumstances are formed by their inner drive to succeed. This drive and this success have a sexual foundation, and readers are certain to see the text as an exploration of the differences between men and women. By ignoring the rules that the other characters follow, Ambrosio and Matilda open themselves to the possibility of an unknown *jouissance*, a limitless pleasure. Inevitably, they define male and female for the text, and readers are attracted to the sexual tension which accompanies their appearance. Their love story was so popular that James Boaden wrote a theatrical adaptation entitled Aurelio_and Miranda in which Matilda is rewritten as the chaste virgin Miranda who redeems and marries the Ambrosio-like Aurelio. This play ran only briefly. Audiences apparently disliked the moral modifications.[24]

If Lewis actually intended any moral purpose for his novel, he was unable to convince critics like Coleridge and Mathias. They recognized that the ostensibly rectifying punishments and rewards at the end of the novel do little to erase the erotic and profane descriptions throughout the text. Instead of leading to moral conclusions, Lewis created characters who define themselves by following their sexual instincts and by defying authority to stop them. Ambrosio establishes a masculine presence not through following a Protestant work ethic or by living up to an aristocratic ideal, but by pursuing his sexual desires and attempting to find that *jouissance* which would return him to a state of sexual bliss with his symbolic mother. This attempt is doomed from the start because it is an ideal that Ambrosio seeks through physical means and because, in Lewis's view, male sexual desire itself is disgusting and corrupting. On the final page, Ambrosio resembles a fallen Prometheus or an exiled Oedipus as "the eagles of the rock tore his flesh piecemeal, and dug out his eyeballs with their crooked beaks" (420). Unchecked, his male sex drive has led him to depravity and defeat, and his punishment demonstrates his failure to fulfill his Promethean promise and the Oedipal horror beneath male desire. Within every man, Lewis suggests, is this sexual monster.

Lewis's villainous monk reflects the troubled masculinity of the eighteenth century. Once the authority of the father is questioned, then questions also arise regarding sexual restraint and the roles of men and women in general. Male characters like Ambrosio, Lovelace, and Manfred are evil because they go too far in ignoring the boundaries of what most readers would consider acceptable behavior. However, their status as individuals in confrontation with a system that restricts and denies them pleasure provides these males with a masculinity that other characters lack. While readers generally find the acts of these villains abhorrent, these same readers may admire the self-sufficiency that the characters display and may even share these characters' desires for an unlimited and unrestricted sexual pleasure outside of societal regulations. Distinguishing between good and bad behavior is not always simple for readers, however, because if everyone has sexual desire, as is portrayed in Lewis's novel, then the difference between villains and heroes is simply a matter of degree. Since sexual desire is so problematic, what is left, according to Lewis, is a dilemma which pits the male against himself in a battle between desire of the female body and love of the mother. In this scenario, it is the mother's love which places limitations on desire and not the father's word, and it is the male who fails because he is unable to contain his desires.

Years after publication of <u>The Monk</u> and toward the end of his life, Lewis wrote "The Isle of Devils," a poem in heroic couplets about a Caliban-type monster who rapes a maiden marooned on his island.

When she escapes the island, ironically rescued by monks, she leaves behind her monster child, and the final scene shows a father holding his infant son, wailing at their loss, then plunging into the sea to their deaths. This image of a son, abandoned by his mother, resembles the circumstances of the character Ambrosio and Lewis himself; however, in this instance, the demonic nature of the son creates a morally ambiguous situation where the mother deserts a demon child. If she stays, she nurtures a monster, but by leaving she ignores her role as mother. In effect, Lewis creates ambiguity by shifting responsibility from the mother to the male child's nature. In this view, the child creates the mother, and, hideous because he is his father's son, the child is unable to preserve the mother-child bond. Instead of an Oedipal conflict between father and son, both males fail to win the woman's love, perhaps because of their very nature as males.

Notes

[1]qtd in Louis F. Peck, A Life of Matthew G. Lewis (Cambridge: Harvard UP, 1961) 170.

[2]Chris Jones, Radical Sensibility: Literature and Ideas in the 1790s (London: Routledge, 1993). Jones sees three trends in sensibility: the potentially radical, the conservative, and the self-indulgent, which only at the end of the century become unraveled and eventually suppressed by anti-Jacobin rhetoric.

[3]Devendra Varma, The Gothic Flame (New York: Russell, 1957) 129; see also Ernest Bernbaum, Guide through the Romantic Movement (New York: Ronald P, 1930) 33-34, which Varma references.

[4]In his discussion of the psychological and social effects of pornography, Mark Bracher, in Lacan, Discourse, and Social Change: A Psychoanalytic Cultural Criticism (Ithaca: Cornell UP, 1993), describes how pornography also operates to exclude love while focusing on desire. In The Monk, this same technique is used to heighten sexual interest, but instead of privileging the penis as phallus, Lewis appears to position the female as the unapproachable phallus. Lewis promotes a difference between the desires of men and women rather than denying it like pornography.

[5]Kenneth W. Graham, afterword, Gothic Fictions: Prohibition / Transgression (New York: AMS P, 1989) 266.

[6]David Punter, The Literature of Terror (New York: Longman, 1980) 92.

[7]Peter Brooks, "Virtue and Terror: The Monk," ELH 40 (1973) 262

[8]Brooks 258.

[9]Sade is quoted in Varma, 150-151; also Graham 260.

[10]Peck 133.

[11]Peck 33.

[12]Peck 123.

[13]Bracher 68.

[14]Matthew G. Lewis, The Monk (New York: Grove Press, 1952) 148; all subsequent references will be to this text.

[15]Kristina Straub, Sexual Suspects: Eighteenth-Century Players and Sexual Ideology (Princeton: Princeton UP, 1992) 19.

[16]See Syndy M. Conger, "Sensibility Restored: Radcliffe's Answer to Lewis's The Monk," Gothic Fictions: Prohibition/Transgression, ed. by Kenneth W. Graham (New York, AMS P, 1989) 113-149, for a discussion of Lewis's use of the sensational as an extension of sensibility. Conger also mentions the apparent influence of Rousseau in Lewis's description of Ambrosio's path to corruption via an improper education.

[17]William Patrick Day, In the Circles of Fear and Desire: A Study of Gothic Fantasy (Chicago: U of Chicago P, 1985); see particularly Day's description of the presence of voyeurism in the Gothic novel, pages 62-69.

[18]Day 121.

[19]Jacqueline Howard, Reading Gothic Fiction: A Bakhtinian Approach (Oxford: Clarendon P, 1994) 203.

[20]Haggerty, "Literature and Homosexuality," 341; Sedgwick, Between Men, 92; and, Bayer-Berenbaum 41.

[21]Louis F. Peck, Matthew Lewis's primary biographer, states flatly "that the statement that Lewis was homosexual, while it would require for confirmation more convincing evidence than has been presented, is impossible to confirm or disprove" 66; however, critics seem inclined to equate him with fellow Gothic novelist William Beckford, who suffered public disgrace from his apparent homosexual activities. John Berryman states, "Lewis was, like William Beckford, homosexual." [See the introduction to The Monk (New York: Grove P, 1952) 23.] The main evidence to support such a conclusion is a journal remark by Byron regarding Lewis's interest in boys and a relationship with a young man in which Lewis provided financial support (see Peck 65). Both of these incidents occurred years after publication of The Monk, however, and neither proves Lewis to be either exclusively or actively homosexual.

[22]Peck 36.

[23]Hume 287.

[24]Peck 31.

CHAPTER VII

GODWIN AND THE NATURE OF POWER

But when, by what test, by what indication does manhood
commence? Physically, by one criterion, legally by another.
Morally by a third, intellectually by a fourth--and all indefinite.

Thomas De Quincey, Autobiography[1]

The varied manifestations of masculinity portrayed by Richardson's Lovelace, Walpole's Manfred, and Lewis's Ambrosio have in common a sexual power that threatens and destroys women. Each of these male characters is a sexual rogue, defining himself by the manner in which he treats women and the way he ignores societal opinion; consequently, the differences between these males and the other male characters in Clarissa, The Castle of Otranto, and The Monk are most apparent in their relationships with female characters. Characters who are contrasted against the villains, like Belford, Theodore, and Lorenzo, protect rather than imprison and terrorize women, and they use their male power to restore the social norm rather than confront it. At stake in these novels, therefore, is not the issue of male power, but what form that male power should take. Inevitably, these protective males negotiate a marriage contract which will allow them access to an appropriately attractive female body, continuation of their family name, and a social harmony equated with happiness, and this use of the marriage contract to perpetuate patriarchal authority can be seen as just another means

197

of subjugating women.[2] At the same time, these images of "successful manhood" represent a difficult standard of masculinity that achieves economic stability, gains political power, and denies sexual desire by replacing but not clearly combining it with love.

This use of marriage as a reward for "morally correct" male behavior overlooks the competitive nature of that behavior and offers a simple solution to what might otherwise be the complex issue of male difference. Marriage, in these novels, solves the problem of male desire by implying that all desires are met and a completeness as well as a form of immortality are created by the wedding of the hero and heroine. In Lacanian terms, marriage operates as the master signifier (S1) which resolves the hysterical discourse ($) caused by the absence of a superintending authority (S1) and the acknowledgment of a lack (a) that the search for pleasure, happiness, or immortality implies. The Gothic novel, in particular, presents anxiety-creating images of castration, which reinforce recognition of this lack (a), in its use of ruined castles and fragmented and decaying bodies and resolves this anxiety only when the villain, often the representative of unleashed male sexual energy, has been annihilated. Endings where the male hero, like Theodore or Lorenzo, does not marry his initial beloved, who is dead, but a woman who replaces her, emphasize the importance of the signifier "marriage" above any considerations of love or desire. The significance of marriage in these novels is not that it unites two individuals who love each other but that it somehow sets things right.

The ostensibly happy marriage at the end of the Gothic narrative alleviates reader anxiety and provides a resolution to the plot; however, this formulaic coupling of young men and women also reduces both genders to a one-dimensional status and creates few individual differences among the characters. For males, this means that while Theodore, Lorenzo, Raymond, or Valencourt and Vivaldi of Ann Radcliffe's The Mysteries of Udolpho or The Italian all appear as exemplary men in comparison to the villains they oppose, they do little to distinguish or define themselves in the course of the novel and succeed mainly because the villain is removed by some other greater force (heavenly, demonic, or institutional). The eighteenth century Gothic novel tends to center around the young heroine, who is the victim or potential victim of male violence,[3] because she represents a sexual object, an object of desire, which the villains and the readers recognize; at the same time, the young heroes are defined only marginally and usually in conjunction with their failure as protectors against the greater force of the villain. The active and defining masculinity which emerges from the Gothic novel always belongs to the villain, but he is also the aggressor and in charge of the fate which awaits him. The male, either as villain or young hero, is seldom examined as the oppressed in the Gothic novel, except perhaps in the work of William Godwin.

Of all the eighteenth century novels labeled "Gothic," Godwin's Caleb Williams stands out as the text most unfairly stigmatized by this categorization,[4] possibly because it does not create the sexual atmosphere generally associated with the genre. Although Godwin was reading Radcliffe's Udolpho while writing Caleb Williams[5] and borrowed the device of a mysterious locked trunk from her Romance of the Forest,[6] he avoided the medieval setting and the supernatural occurrences found in the earlier novels of horror. While he explores themes common to the Gothic like confinement and the abuse of power, Godwin was no doubt influenced more heavily by the philosophical and picaresque novels of his close friend Thomas Holcroft, whose Anna St. Ives was published in 1792, than by Otranto or Udolpho. During this time, Godwin's conversations with Holcroft provided him with many of the ideas which would appear in his most significant works, Enquiry Concerning Political Justice and Caleb Williams, and Holcroft is credited with having had "the greatest effect on Godwin during the composition of Political Justice."[7]

Published in 1794, one year after Godwin's famous philosophical and political treatise, Caleb Williams was written not just to entertain but to provide, as Godwin discloses in his first Preface, "a general review of the modes of domestic and unrecorded despotism, by which man becomes the destroyer of man."[8] In Political Justice, Godwin argues for human perfectibility and the correspondent demise of government,[9] and in Caleb Williams he promotes these same ideas by demonstrating many of the human and institutional errors that prevent men from achieving happiness. Originally entitled Things as They Are, Godwin's novel was an attempt to demonstrate his newly introduced philosophical ideas "to persons, whom books of philosophy and science are never likely to reach."[10] Although he succeeded in creating a text which appealed to a significant number of readers, his success in using a popular novel to promote his philosophy appears limited.

Elizabeth Inchbald's concern that the popularity of the novel would be damaged by its radicalism proved unfounded.[11] More disturbing to Godwin was his reader's avoidance of the philosophical message in the course of what they discovered to be an entertaining reading experience. Almost forty years after his novel's publication, Godwin expressed disappointment at having had Caleb Williams received as "a book to amuse boys and girls in their vacant hours, a story to be gobbled up by them, swallowed in a pusillanimous and untainted mood, without chewing and digestion."[12] Critics have similarly had difficulty in finding an approach which acknowledges both Godwin's proposed philosophical purposes and the resultant work of fiction. While <u>Caleb Williams</u> has been given historical significance by those who connect it to "the development of the detective novel, the political novel, the philosophical novel, the psychological thriller and the novel of pursuit,"[13] the novel's philosophical content has been somehow subordinated to its machinery, and that machinery, generally classified as "Gothic," has placed Godwin's novel outside of the canon and into this category of popular fiction.

At the same time, however, critics of the Gothic novel, failing to find many of the devices prevalent in the majority of Gothic texts, place <u>Caleb Williams</u> at the margin of their studies. Perhaps Edith Birkhead established this practice by stating in her landmark early work, <u>The Tale of Terror</u>, that Godwin "had neither the gift nor the inclination to conjure with Gothic properties;"[14] nevertheless, whether subsequent critics have followed her lead or arrived at a similar estimate on their own, <u>Caleb Williams</u> "has always been considered only 'borderline' Gothic."[15] Thus, having had its message reduced by its association with a group of texts cast out of the traditional canon, the attention paid to Godwin's novel has suffered further diminution by its peripheral relationship to the Gothic genre. Therefore, in spite of its immense immediate success,[16] <u>Caleb Williams</u> has generated, with Godwin's other writings, "no organized body of followers,"[17] and has generally been excluded from discussions about important eighteenth century fiction.

Probably the most active recent commentator on Godwin's work, Kenneth W. Graham, suggests that this relative obscurity extends from a prejudice against Godwin's political view developed during the politically conservative period which began shortly after the publication of his two greatest works.[18] Godwin's principal biographer, Peter H. Marshall, shares this view. "It was Godwin's misfortune," according to Marshall, "to have his name closely linked to the

French Revolution," and because of this association, Godwin "was at first vilified and then rapidly forgotten."[19] While I do not wish to take up this particular cause and all of its potential complexity, I see a connection between Graham's and Marshall's remarks regarding prejudice and the use of Gothic categorization to outlaw or restrict certain texts. In this case, <u>Caleb Williams</u> shares little in common in terms of theme, plot, or setting with any of the other major works generally called Gothic. Only in the characterization of men who terrorize each other and in the choice of words like demon, spectre, devil, ghost, chimera, and basilisk to describe otherwise realistic personages does <u>Caleb Williams</u> adopt traditionally Gothic characteristics.[20] As R. D. Spector points out, critics have always been more likely to read this text as a socio-political novel,[21] and until the twentieth century the novel's Gothic connection was largely ignored. This late stigmatization as Gothic follows a century of reviews which generally focus negatively upon "Godwin's philosophy or his "moral principles" while offering only limited commentary on "Godwin's fictional abilities."[22] It is not surprising perhaps that this exiled novel should inevitably be consigned to the lower levels of the generic strata.

Currently, Godwin's oppositional ideology[23] is being reevaluated because of its emphasis on the necessity of social change at a time when the "modern capitalist, industrial society"[24] was created. In conjunction with this renewed interest in the ingenuity of Godwin's radical thought, <u>Caleb Williams</u>, with its focus on male behavior and the evils of power, needs to be reconsidered as both a socio-political and a Gothic novel. Because Godwin's male characters struggle to define themselves and ultimately prove to be powerless, they portray a unique masculinity which demonstrates the futility of the male desire for phallic power. The villains, for Godwin, are not males whose desires drive them to commit heinous crimes, but institutions which pit men against each other and perpetuate a competition that harms everyone. Being a man is important for the three main male characters, Caleb, Falkland, and Tyrrel, and because they associate manhood with a type of power, each wrongly sees the others as adversaries. The terror in Caleb Williams occurs, in part, because of their efforts to play out those manly roles which they have been provided by their education, and it is their failure to see the truth beneath the fallacy of an aggressive manhood which causes each of them misery.

The story is told in three very distinct volumes and involves no ghosts, castles, or supernatural phenomena. Volume I begins with Caleb's first person narration but quickly changes to the third person as Caleb retells Falkland's history as told to him by Mr. Collins, Caleb's mentor. This history discloses Falkland's multiple confrontations with Tyrrel, like Falkland a local squire, but, unlike Falkland, an "arrogant" "tyrannical," and "insolent" (19) bully. Tyrrel unfairly persecutes his tenants, the Hawkinses, and eventually causes his cousin and ward, Emily Melville, to escape from his estate and die when he has her unjustly imprisoned. Before she dies, Falkland saves Emily's life from a fire and fortuitously prevents her rape by Grimes, a coarse local rustic to whom Tyrrel has promised Emily in marriage. Volume I ends when, after a public altercation in which Tyrrel physically humiliates Falkland, Tyrrel is killed on his way home. The unknown assailant is first thought to be Falkland; however, after he is exonerated and evidence implicating the Hawkinses is found, they are executed for the murder. Because he believes, above all else, in the importance of honor, Falkland, meanwhile, apparently has never recovered from his public humiliation.

Volume II covers the time Caleb, an orphan who is made secretary to Falkland, spends within the enclosed sphere of Falkland's direct influence. Caleb's curiosity regarding Falkland's dejected demeanor leads him to spy on his master, and his relentless probing eventually causes Falkland to confess that he killed Tyrrel. After this revelation, Falkland tells Caleb that he can never again live outside of Falkland's control, and Caleb immediately begins his attempts to escape. When Mr. Forester, Falkland's half-brother, befriends Caleb, Caleb tries to use this connection to free himself from Falkland. This backfires, however, as Falkland accuses Caleb of stealing and plants evidence on him to support these accusations. Imprisoned for this crime, Caleb ingeniously attempts two escapes and finally succeeds at the end of the volume.

The third and final volume contains Caleb's adventures beyond Falkland's immediate control, but shows how his apparent freedom outside the prison walls is an illusion because Caleb is constantly in fear of discovery and in need of a financial means of survival. During this time, Caleb hides himself by falling in with a group of bandits and by impersonating a beggar, an Irishman, a Jew, and a hunchback. Though he does not join the bandits in the commission of their crimes, he accepts a share of their stolen wealth, and, later, he finds employment as a hack writer. At last, however, the bounty hunter Gines (Jones in the original edition) finds him and brings him to the magistrate. Caleb finally reveals Falkland's secret, which he has kept throughout his persecution, but the magistrate does not believe him. Subsequently, however, when Caleb's prosecutors fail to show for his trial, he is set free. When Falkland's agent Gines continues to follow Caleb and ruin his name, Caleb once again accuses Falkland of the murder of Tyrrel and a hearing is set. At the hearing Caleb and Falkland see the truth in each other's positions and both regret their behavior. Falkland dies three days later, and Caleb closes the novel with the self-realization that he will always be miserable because he ruined so great a man.

Undisputedly, <u>Caleb Williams</u> was tremendously popular in its own time. "Few books made a greater impression on their first appearance."[25] Within three years of its initial publication, <u>Things as They Are; or, the Adventures of Caleb Williams</u> had been published in three British editions and three French and two German translations. Irish and American editions appeared in 1795.[26] In his study of British reviews from 1788-1802, Derek Roper concludes that <u>Caleb Williams</u> was probably "[t]he most powerful novel written during this period,"[27] Graham states assertively, "[t]here is little doubt that [Godwin's 1794 novel] was widely read and broadly influential,"[28] and George Sherburn credits this work with being "certainly the first impressive tragic novel since Richardson's <u>Clarissa</u>."[29]

Nevertheless, given the extent to which Godwin and his novel have been said to have affected all of the major Romantic poets[30] and influenced the development of a variety of fictional genres, the significance of this work remains "to a considerable degree un-avowed,"[31] and <u>Caleb Williams</u> has been relatively ignored. Only recently have critics found a multiplicity of approaches to a text whose complex narrative structure and political purposes create an ambiguity which opens the door to debate. Since the discovery by D. Gilbert Dumas of an earlier ending to the novel which shows Caleb's attempt at prosecution leading only to reimprisonment and insanity,[32] these debates have included a discussion of the "conflict between Godwin the novelist and Godwin the philosopher,"[33] and have questioned whether <u>Caleb Williams</u> fulfilled its author's stated socio-political intentions.[34] Godwin's late claims, published almost forty years after this novel that he began in the third person and changed to the first person while writing the three volumes in reverse order from last to first[35] have also produced questions about the reliability of the author as well as the narrator. As Karl Simms points out, Godwin and Caleb share in their textual efforts to bring the truth to light, but both mix fiction and truth and, therefore, create doubts in the minds of their readers.[36] Ironically, the fact that "there is a wealth of documentary evidence surrounding the composition and intention of <u>William Godwin's Caleb Williams, or Things as They Are</u>" only leads critics to conclude that we cannot "take Godwin's own statements too literally" because "such an abundance of material can lead us into obvious trouble."[37] However, the end result of all this ambiguity is the lack of anything approaching a consistent reading.

While many critics agree that <u>Caleb Williams</u> was significantly influential with contemporary readers, the nature of the novel's impact on those readers remains in question. Whether the novel is viewed as an exploration of the psychological consequences of the political status quo of Godwin's time or the political consequences of the behavior of men who fail to confront the psychological truths of their condition, <u>Caleb Williams</u> has resisted an interpretation which examines both the aspects of Caleb's mental torment and the tyrannizing nature of the political apparatus. In Mitzi Myers' words, "The mutually exclusive political and psychological interpretations identify and clarify two important aspects of <u>CW</u>, but the interdependence of the understanding and the imagination [which she notes that Hazlitt saw in Godwin's novel] remains obscured by divergent critical overemphases."[38] Without a more comprehensive analysis, <u>Caleb Williams</u> cannot be fully understood from the perspective of its readership. After all, for readers this is a mystery novel, and their interest is engaged by a sequence of surprising events which have reasonable cause and effect explanations, some psychologically-based and some politically-motivated.

Reconciling the political and psychological forces at work in the novel has proved difficult. Myers' attempt to re-label Godwin's political problems as "essentially moral problems"[39] overlooks the dangerous political nature of Godwin's external circumstances, which caused him to withhold the potentially inflammatory Preface from the original edition. Furthermore, while her approach stresses the moral lessons that Caleb learns while advancing first into and then away from "selfish egoism,"[40] she fails to account for the ambiguity that has made the ending so problematic. For Don Locke, for example, <u>Caleb Williams</u> seems to endorse aristocratic values, "implying that the intrinsic worth of a Falkland can survive even the most malevolent actions." "Godwin's moral," Locke states, "is one thing; but the tendency of his book, its actual effect of the reader, seems quite another." [41]

Because Myers reads the book with her eye on the internal changes in the character of Caleb and Locke evaluates the ending based on the external results to the characters, each reaches significantly different conclusions. If neither is guilty of a major misreading, both can be correct only if a third reading discloses a heretofore undiscussed common ground between the psychological and the political. This more coherent reading of <u>Caleb Williams</u> demands that readers reject the mind/body split and see both mind and body unifiedly oppressed by a misguided way of thinking and the necessarily corrupted institutions which pit men against each other.

In <u>Political Justice</u>, Godwin makes clear that he sees no distinction between moral (individual and psychical) and political (social) functions. Although others "have considered the virtues and pleasures of mankind as essentially independent of civil policy," and "have treated morality and personal happiness as one science and politics as a different one,"[42] Godwin combines the two and gives them a common goal: the pursuit of pleasure, or happiness. While, in <u>Caleb Williams</u>, Godwin can be viewed as "attacking the practices and ideology of aristocratic and patrician culture,"[43] or the system of institutions, he is also, as he does in <u>Political Justice</u>, exploring "the subtlety of the human mind"[44] and the manner in which "sound reasoning and truth, when adequately communicated, must always be victorious over error."[45] What must change, in Godwin's view, are not the institutions in themselves, but the perspectives of men. When men, through the use of reason, attain the understanding necessary to recognize the benefits of embracing their natural virtues, these institutions, which are corrupt by nature, will dissolve.

In <u>Political Justice</u>, things are described as they are because men do not recognize the advantages of truth or the pleasures of virtue, but instead operate out of "mercenary self-interest"[46] and have their characters prescribed by political institutions which encourage "a servile and corrupt spirit."[47] A man, ignorant of his circumstances, can only fall victim to the conditions under which he is raised.

> The best that can be expected, is that he should return at last to sobriety and truth, with a mind debilitated and relaxed by repeated errors, and a moral constitution in which seeds of degeneracy have been deeply and extensively sown.[48]

Under the doctrine of necessity, "[m]an is in reality a passive and not an active being," and this allows for an understanding of the "real antecedents"[49] for man's immoral behavior, those social and political institutions that men pay homage to and put their faith in.

In <u>Caleb Williams</u>, Godwin's message is that corrupt political structures are supported by a reluctance of men to see the truth, or things as they are. The manner in which the characters view and react to each other is fixed by not only their social or physical position but also by the manner in which they perceive and reason. The patterns of behavior that the primary male characters enact have to a degree been determined by the conditions of their social upbringing, a type of dark necessity which casts each in a role against the other. However, Godwin was also an idealist who believed in the perfectibility of mankind, so "things as they are" are not things as they have to be, nor, in his optimistic view, as they will be. The tragic conclusion of the novel results from Caleb's and Falkland's inability to recognize the part they play in maintaining the system, even while that system destroys them, but the reader is expected to reconsider their roles and to rethink their seemingly reasonable actions.

Falkland, Caleb, and Tyrrel act repeatedly in their own self-interest and suffer because they do not have the "disinterestedness" (376) and fortitude necessary to step away from the observations they have been taught to make and to enjoy pleasure, endure pain, and face the truth of their condition. Only in the revised ending does Caleb realize that he should have "opened [his] heart to Mr. Falkland" (374) and Falkland understand the evils he has perpetrated "to protect [himself] from the prejudice of [his] species" (376). The earlier, unpublished ending does not contain these self-revelations, and though it completes the pattern of oppression with Caleb's insanity, it less clearly relates Godwin's moral lesson because the main characters do not openly recognize and acknowledge their part in their own disintegration. More consistent with the philosophy of Political Justice, the final, published ending shows that Falkland and Caleb "have been slaves to their limited moral vision and courage,"[50] and they share responsibility for the consequences which place them both in misery.

Man against man, as Godwin indicates in the Preface, they destroy each other, but they do so because they fear the other's power and believe in the institutions which surround them rather than in their inner tendency toward human sympathy and benevolent action. Both use the legal system in an attempt to obtain justice instead of confronting each other honestly and sincerely. At the end of the novel, the discovery of the failure of this system and the immorality of the selfish need to best the other man results in a new masculinity in the form of Caleb's "manly story" (376), which preferences a concern for others above "an overweening regard" for self. This masculinity rejects "the corrupt wilderness of human society" and the societal hierarchies that create and promote an atmosphere of "jealousy and inexorable precaution," and embraces a philosophy of openness, benevolence, and a denial of self-interest. Readers, who like Caleb anticipate his liberation "if the guilt of Falkland [is] established" (377), must reexamine the events of the novel not as a contest between the relentless aristocrat and the cunning and elusive narrator, but as a futile game played by two misguided men.

Whether or not casual readers, the "boys and girls" of Godwin's plaintive remembrance of his novel's reception, conduct such a reexamination seems suspect. Critical commentary has yet to decide on the success of the revised ending,[51] and critics, like Locke, find a "fundamental difficulty" in assigning the "real moral"[52] of Caleb Williams because they recognize the reader's attraction to either the narrative voice of Caleb, which during the final confrontation becomes god-like according to Rudolf Storch,[53] or to "the intrinsic worth of Falkland."[54] Though the ending attempts to show that no man wins, or finds pleasure, by competing with other men, the novel is successful because the remainder of the narrative involves the reader in that competition; consequently, the reader demands an unambiguous resolution and may or may not believe "Caleb's [pejorative] opinion of himself,"[55] or that his treatment of Falkland is justified.[56] In other words, in spite of Godwin's rewriting and philosophical position, readers continue to insist on choosing a winner in the Caleb/Falkland battle.

The point of the text, however, is that there is no winner in this personal war between two males. No matter whether readers see the power relationships in Caleb Williams as resolved in the end or not, those relationships reveal the nature of power as practiced by men upon each other. Power, in this sense, is both political and psychological, as one man struggles to best another in an effort to prove his own definition of man to be the correct one. Godwin challenges the reader to pick the best man, or symbol of masculinity, in his descriptions of and distinctions among the male characters, but his ending shows that no man wins in direct competition with the others. Because, under the doctrine of necessity, no man is entirely at fault for who he is, the descriptions of the characters go beyond stereotyping and attempt to explore the cause and effect of human interaction. Tyrrel, therefore, is not just a brute or a stereotypical country squire; he is a complex individual whose actions have their roots in his upbringing and the treatment he receives from his neighbors prior to Falkland's return to the community. As the recipient of a type of social determination, he is no more responsible for the conflict which follows than Falkland.

The original quarrel between Falkland and Tyrrel which sets in motion the events of the novel is created by the irreconcilable differences in the two men's perspectives, and those perspectives are understood by examining their backgrounds. In terms of their inherited economic position, the two are male equals, but their contrasting physical stature and early training creates antipodal differences in their characters. Tyrrel is "muscular and sturdy" and "his form might have been selected by a painter as a model for that hero of antiquity, whose prowess consisted in felling an ox with his fist, and devouring him at a meal" (19). Overindulged by his mother, "a woman of narrow capacity" (18), Tyrrel develops into an insolent ruffian who has a unrefined, sarcastic wit; however, he excels at this and becomes the grand master of all such men who gather at a weekly assembly. He is also not without innate positive qualities as he occasionally shows "affableness and familiarity" and beneath his rough speech is "a rich, but undisciplined imagination" (20).

As a foil for Falkland, Tyrrel is established as an accomplished tyrant in the physical domain, but he earns this position by surpassing other men, and his masculinity is further verified by the reaction of young women. "Every daughter regarded his athletic form and his acknowledged prowess with a favourable eye" (21). Even though he is a brute, he is a superior male in the eyes of women, and even this misconception has its antecedent cause: "women are taught early to look for [a physically intimidating protector] in the male sex" (21). Guided by his mother, honored by other men, and sexually coveted by women, Tyrrel is the fulfillment of other people's desires. He also represents a physical masculinity which appears out of place in Godwin's picture of a modern world. His "untamed" nature quickly loses favor in the community when Falkland returns after a long absence in Italy and provides a "polished" alternative model of male conduct.

Falkland, in contrast to Tyrrel, is described as small in stature, "with an extreme delicacy of form and appearance" (5). As if to combat the possible readings of effeminacy in this description, Godwin makes certain of Falkland's masculinity by enhancing female reactions. Falkland is "favoured and admired by the softer sex" (11), and "his polished manners were peculiarly in harmony with feminine delicacy" (22). Furthermore, he is "refined without foppery" and "elegant without effeminacy!" (23). Shortly after his return, Falkland's advantages over Tyrrel have been noted by the women and men of the community and Tyrrel finds himself ignored by his former companions. In other words, Falkland's masculinity receives preference over Tyrrel's brutish male behavior.

In this masculinity contest, neither male can accept the other's contrasting position, and aggression and hostility necessarily ensue. Each man's identity requires him to reject the other. For Tyrrel that identity involves a strong, physical image which, combined with an aggressive nature, symbolizes 'man'. For Falkland, male identity has nothing to do with physical stature, but requires "a temper perpetually alive to the sentiments of birth and honour," which conforms to a "model of heroism" (11) that he has learned from reading books about chivalry and romance. While readers are expected to see Falkland initially as "a being of a superior order" (7), not only to Tyrrel but to all the other characters as well, Tyrrel's argument that Falkland uses books and language to adapt "to his miserable [diminutive] condition" (22) is an interesting one and not without foundation. Both men appear, after all, to seek the same recognition in the community. Although Falkland's "dignity," "affability," and "attention to the happiness of others" (23), set him above Tyrrel in the view of the local populace (and the reader), Falkland's concern for honor, or public esteem, creates questions about his motives. His rigid adherence to a code of conduct which provides him a symbolic male identity makes him no less culpable than Tyrrel for the tragic events which follow.

Tyrrel's belief in an imaginary masculinity, or one based on the image of a physically dominant male, clashes with Falkland's symbolic concept of a manhood related metonymically to the signifier 'honor', but they share the presupposition that a superior male exists. Godwin himself proposed a four-tiered hierarchy in a revised edition of Political Justice published in 1796, and Tyrrel appears to belong to Godwin's second level, "men of rank, fortune and dissipation,"[57] while Falkland seemingly possesses the potential to be the highest form of man, "the man of benevolence."[58] However, according to Godwin's theory, this fourth level of man transcends his own interests and endeavors to promote others, to "elevate every man to all true wisdom," and thereby to eventually realize "the true equalization of mankind."[59] Godwin's purpose, therefore, was not to differentiate between classes, but to show that classes exist which prevent happiness and that real happiness would come to pass when all men reached the highest level of disinterestedness in self and concern for others. Falkland subsequently fails to embody Godwin's "man of benevolence" because he allows his own self-interest, his concern for honor, to dictate his actions. Rather than relying on his predisposition toward virtuous acts, Falkland builds a system of signifiers which are more important to him than his acts themselves. He mistakenly, according to Godwin's philosophy, adopts a male identity which inflexibly defends itself against attacks to those signifiers and which invariably implies its own superiority and, by doing so, creates its own hierarchy.

The confrontations between Tyrrel and Falkland represent the conflict between two types of male power, and each male character needs to prove superiority in order to maintain a masculine identity constructed upon the belief that a hierarchical order exists. At stake is not only who is the better man, but who embodies the signifier 'man' itself. To lose such a battle is not to be diminished but to be castrated. Not coincidentally, their initial collision takes place in connection to a woman, a common site for male power struggles. When Miss Hardingham, a young woman for whom Tyrrel's "general preference" was "notorious" (24), attempts to make Tyrrel jealous by promising the dance of the evening at a village assembly to an unaware Falkland, the exchange between the two men indicates the seriousness of their differences. Tyrrel claims ownership of Miss Hardingham and her affections, and while Falkland disclaims interest in such matters, he refuses to yield his position as her escort. Their dialogue demonstrates the connection between property rights and masculinity and ends when Falkland declares, "[N]o man shall prevent my asserting that, to which I have once acquired a claim!" (25). Since this battle is being waged with words and not physical acts, it is no surprise that Falkland defeats Tyrrel, and the result has implications about the comparative masculinity of the two men. After Falkland's declaration, "the ferociousness of his antagonist subside[s] into impotence," and Tyrrel walks away "without answering a word" (25). Emasculated by Falkland's words, Tyrrel can only brood over "this rebellion against his authority" (26) and plot revenge. This incident has marked him as Falkland's inferior, an untenable position given his belief in his own superior masculinity, and he must either strike back or forfeit his manhood.

Until his final encounter with Falkland, Tyrrel struggles to reestablish his male authority, but the community's increasing admiration for Falkland prevents this. Tyrrel's persecution of his cousin Emily occurs because she acquires an affection for his male rival, and his injustice toward the Hawkinses also has its roots in his uneasy masculinity. Hawkins' refusal to send his son into service with Tyrrel turns an otherwise generous act on the part of Tyrrel into a question of authority. Their argument is punctuated by Tyrrel's astonishment that the "lord of the manor" (82) could be questioned, and his male identity, dependent upon that authority and already injured by Falkland, cannot suffer the further damage of Hawkins's refusal. When Tyrrel rhetorically questions how "a rascal" like Hawkins can "pretend to beard the lord of the manor" (81), he restates the frustration he feels in his efforts to maintain his manhood. Only an inevitable showdown with Falkland can restore his identity.

Falkland, although ostensibly the peacemaker, does little to discourage this final confrontation. When he visits Tyrrel in an effort to set aside their differences, Falkland cannot hide his belief in his own superiority. During his visit, he is described as having "an apparent loftiness in his manner, that [i]s calculated to irritate" (34); he is not just a passive recipient in this duel of masculinities, but a co-instigator. Tyrrel categorizes Falkland's behavior as his "bullying airs" (108), and Falkland resembles Tyrrel in the forcefulness and resoluteness he uses to get the respect of the community which he desires. While their methods differ, the two men share the same desires and sense of purpose.

When Tyrrel physically assaults Falkland, he restores his own masculine position and destroys Falkland's. His attack overwhelms Falkland and shows how completely Falkland is his physical inferior. After knocking Falkland down twice, Tyrrel kicks his prostrate body and then prepares to drag the apparently helpless Falkland along the floor. Only the intercession of other gentlemen prevents Falkland from suffering further indignities. Although Tyrrel's violence is contemptible, his aggression has been necessitated by the destruction caused by Falkland's alternative version of manhood on Tyrrel's image of masculinity. Given his belief system, Tyrrel's physical mastery of Falkland is necessary to avoid the obliteration of his male identity. Likewise, to Falkland, for whom "disgrace was worse than death," "this complication of ignominy, base, humiliating and public" (110) marks his symbolic death, or, in other words, the end of his link to the signifier 'honor'. Metonymically, to be 'Falkland' is to be 'a man' which means to have 'honor'. Losing 'honor' means losing self; therefore, this symbolic death for Falkland is worse than real, physical death, and he reacts by wishing "for annihilation" and "eternal oblivion" (110).

Falkland's honor and identity can never be restored, but he reduces Tyrrel in the only way he can: he kills him. Tyrrel's physical image is thus removed and Tyrrel's physical authority is eliminated, but Falkland's own version of masculine power has already been proved impotent. For the remainder of the text until he is "conquered" (376) by the truth of Caleb's confession, Falkland will attempt to superficially maintain an image of an honorable man, but his symbolic link to 'honor' has been severed and cannot be reattached. His redemption at the end occurs not by regaining the honor which he had unwisely identified with, but by gaining the understanding that the only virtue worth cultivating is that which arises from within and has nothing to do with the societal forces which govern from outside. Instead of heeding the words of Mr. Collins, "My honour is in my own keeping, beyond the reach of all mankind" (113), Falkland has wrongly concerned himself with the opinion of the world. In an effort to "protect" himself from the "prejudice" of the human "species" (376), Falkland constructs a fictional exterior and this self-interested position keeps him from realizing his potential as Godwin's "man of benevolence." Only when Falkland "bless [es] the hand that wounds [him]"(376) does he recognize his true greatness, a recognition that Caleb then shares. In effect, Falkland tyrannically hounds Caleb to maintain a false image of honor and ignores the "sublime" "intellectual powers" and "godlike ambition" which provide him with a virtuous inner nature which is superior to the honorable image which he would construct.

Those readers who see Falkland triumphing at the end no doubt read the recognition of this inner virtue as evidence of his ultimately superior nature; however, Falkland never actually recovers from his loss of honor, and the lesson he learns just before he dies serves only as a reminder of his wasted existence. This is the tragedy of things as they are. Godwin's optimistic belief in man's essential goodness coincides with his belief that this goodness is tainted by the world's fictions. The only way to avoid these corrupting influences is to deal with others truthfully without a desire for physical mastery (the Imaginary register) like Tyrrel or symbolic significance (the Symbolic register) like Falkland. Caleb's reckoning at the end similarly expresses his acknowledgment of the futility of his efforts to discover the truth about Falkland from sources other than Falkland and to escape from this corrupted world once he is imbricated in it.

If Caleb learns a moral lesson, he does so not by advancing from "innocence to experience,"[60] as Gerald Barker contends, but by finally facing Falkland and confronting the truth which was always in front of him. While Caleb may reach this point out of a desperation caused by his alienation from human contact,[61] his lesson is learned during the final hearing and not prior to it. His last narrative remarks before the final chapter indicate that he still places more importance on his self-interested fear of Falkland than on the need to confront Falkland with the truth. During his chance meeting with Mr. Collins, Caleb considers what Collins's help might mean:

> Might not Mr. Falkland reduce him to a condition as wretched and low as mine? After all, was it not vice in me to desire to involve another man in my sufferings? If I regarded them as intolerable, this was still an additional reason why I should bear them alone. (360)

Although Caleb's concern for Collins can be seen as a redeeming feature of an otherwise solipsistic passage, that concern is shown to be rhetorical when Collins subsequently offers to assist Caleb (if possible), and Caleb, in spite of the possible consequences to Collins, does not reject this assistance. Only later, when Caleb comes face to face with the corpse-like Falkland, does he put his own self-interests aside and show such an honest remorse that he brings his auditors to tears.

Of course, Caleb's moment of revelation is also Falkland's, and the mutuality of this epiphanic self-discovery calls attention to a similarity between the two men which has existed throughout the narrative. Critics have seen the two characters as "aspects of one and the same soul,"[62] or "doubles,"[63] and a sound comparison can be made between Caleb's attempt to restore his reputation and Falkland's attempt to retain his.[64] Nevertheless, Caleb defines himself differently than Falkland, and though he lacks the wealth of Falkland or Tyrrel, he offers his own form of masculine power. Whether or not Caleb "represents the artisans like Thomas Paine and Francis Place who were beginning to assert their rights"[65] or is a harbinger "of a brave new world in which the strongest, and not the most honorable, will rule,"[66] he clearly belongs not only to a different class of men in the Marxist sense, but also a different class of mankind in the Godwinian sense. Although his particular rank is not mentioned in Political Justice, where Godwin lists the unconscious laborer, the man of rank and dissipation, the man of taste and liberal accomplishments, and the man of benevolence, Caleb appears to represent that man who has the capacity to rise above his class with the aid of a man such as Falkland, the potential man of benevolence.[67] However, Falkland's defensiveness, created by his guilt, his terrible secret, and his lost honor, prevents him from promoting Caleb's happiness and, instead, manifests itself in a tyrannical control over Caleb's body, which, in turn, leads Caleb into duplicitous actions.

These actions develop Caleb's primary characteristic: his ability to analyze and adapt to the variety of novel situations he is presented with during his adventures. When he overhears his reputation as the notorious criminal Kit Williams, a man who is "loved" for "his cleverness" (275), he cannot help but feel proud of his accomplishments. Paradoxically, he acquires a notoriety of which many are aware at the same time that he loses a reputation (his good name) about which few cared. The distorted legend of Kit Williams, however, has little connection to the lived reality of Caleb Williams, and there is irony in the fact that men both love and hate Kit, or Caleb, without knowing him. Still, he is proud of his exploits and the knowledge that "when I am no more, my fame shall still survive" (327). After all, the novel represents his retelling of those exploits, and, until the final chapter which occurs outside the frame of the rest of the text, he argues for a form of entrepreneurial male power that succeeds by outwitting authority.

He is not a mirror of Falkland but a different kind of man who relies upon his own ingenuity to establish his identity. When Caleb states, "I was not born indeed to the possession of hereditary wealth; but I had a better inheritance, an enterprising mind, an inquisitive spirit, a liberal ambition" (296), he proudly differentiates himself from Falkland and points out his own superior qualities. His skeptical nature prevents him from accepting Collins's conclusions about Falkland's innocence, and while he "worship[s]" Falkland as a "being of a superior nature" (139), his penetrating questions and irresponsible searches demonstrate that he places no value on Falkland's societal status. Donald R. Wehrs has said that Caleb questions the traditional narrative provided by Collins and as a "counter-hegemonic critic,"[68] he deconstructs that narrative, but Caleb's anti-authority stance requires that hegemonic discourse and, consequently, participates in that discourse. It is the "indistinct apprehension of something arbitrary and tyrannical in the prohibition" which lures him to "do what is forbidden" (124), and his identity is formed by cynicism, disagreement, and evasion. This identity, however, depends upon Falkland's presence in his life because without an authority to question, defy, or even emulate, Caleb's powers of mind, spirit, and ambition would have no outlet.

By not living up to his potential as a man of benevolence, Falkland fails Caleb and misleads him; however, Caleb's own aggressive nature causes Falkland to become defensive and to exercise his power as lord of the manor. Their contest of wills pits Caleb's desire for "the liberty of acting as I pleased" (168) against Falkland's desire to control him and maintain an honorable image, but, unlike the earlier Falkland/Tyrrel confrontation, both characters seem drawn to this conflict. Caleb has "an almost sexually intense passion to know [Falkland's secret], and takes "sadistic delight in spying on his master,"[69] and Falkland appears to desire Caleb's interest when he permits Caleb to ask poignant questions and to stay near him in spite of his inquisitiveness. The relationship between Caleb and Falkland, as John Bender has pointed out, is profoundly sexual and sado-masochistic[70] in nature, and the sexual quality of their relationship is reproduced in the competition between the two ideologies they embrace and the power they wield. Falkland relies on legal, economic, and social forces to limit and discredit his adversary and tells Caleb, "all your weapons are impotent" (177); at the same time, Caleb uses ingenuity and disguise to outwit Falkland and later states, "I exult . . . over the impotence of my persecutor" (216). Rather than attempting to discuss differences, each man utilizes the male power he believes he commands, and each man uses the other to prove the authority of his power and the relative insignificance of his adversary's.

Thus, the conflict between Caleb and Falkland resembles the Tyrrel/Falkland showdown in the importance each character gives to besting the individual he identifies as his opponent. For each of these males, proving himself superior to this 'other' man is linked to his identity, and this identity has a particularly sexual or masculine significance. Masculinity is linked to conquest for the economic equals, Tyrrel and Falkland, but Caleb enjoys his relationship to power and creates his own male identity through this relationship. Tyrrel's and Falkland's differing emphases on the imaginary and the symbolic are unimportant to Caleb, who defines himself in contrast to the world of both Tyrrel and Falkland. Since the two members of the landed gentry have, as I discussed earlier, misled themselves into believing in their particular forms of manhood, Caleb's oppositional position should allow him to avoid the pitfalls of this power struggle and place a greater significance on human relationships. However, his desire to possess a power over Falkland locates him in the midst of this contest for supremacy and precludes him from the pleasure of human contact, like that which he temporarily experiences in his relationship with the motherly Laura and her family. While Caleb succeeds in proving himself to be a man, he ends up as miserable and alone as Tyrrel and Falkland.

For Caleb, the success of his mental prowess signifies manhood and survival, and the two words become synonymous for him. Accosted by an agent for Falkland, he must size up his male opponent:

> I remarked that my enemy was alone; and I believed that, man to man, I might reasonably hope to get the better of him, either by the firmness of my determination, or the subtlety of my invention. (183)

Later, he performs admirably when physically defending himself from a gang of robbers, and when struck by a cutlass, he saves himself by using his shirt as a bandage. Pursued by Gines, he asks rhetorically, "Why, man to man, may I not by the powers of my mind attain the ascendancy over him?" (355). Being the better man means retaining his liberty and, considering the expected outcome of the judicial proceedings, staying alive. In other words, what is usually read as a test of Caleb's survival skills can also be read as a trial of his masculinity. In this way, Caleb resembles Falkland and Tyrrel in his need to prove his male identity, but, in the end, his efforts, like theirs, only lead him to misery. Because Caleb endures, readers like Myers sometimes see the outcome of Caleb's adventures as a triumph for him; however, the ending reveals that Caleb's belief in the power of ingenuity is as misguided as Falkland's belief in honor and aristocratic authority or Tyrrel's belief in physical power. In the end, Tyrrel is physically murdered, Falkland dies dishonored, and Caleb discovers that all of his ingenuity has been misdirected.

In contrast to these doomed masculinities, Godwin offers alternatives in the text which allow for comparison to the main male characters. Mr. Clare, a revered poet who has retired to the rural community, can be considered the "true embodiment of Godwin's conception of virtue,"[71] a man of "perfect wisdom and understanding,"[72] and it is he who, on his deathbed, advises Falkland to guard against the "impatience of imagined dishonour" (39). The venerable Mr. Collins also offers philosophical wisdom when he states Godwin's concept of necessity to Caleb:

> I regard you as vicious; but I do not consider the vicious as proper objects of indignation and scorn. I consider you as a machine: you are not constituted, I am afraid, to be greatly useful to your fellow men; but you did not make yourself; you are just what circumstances irresistibly compelled you to be. I am sorry for your ill properties; but I entertain no enmity against you, nothing but benevolence. (360)

Collins and Clare represent different ways of approaching the struggle for male power. Though Collins fails to see Falkland's faults, he recognizes the liberality and goodness of the man and sees no reason to question whether Falkland murdered Tyrrel or not. Just as Clare has no awareness of the honor which the community bestows upon him, Collins indicates to Caleb that true innocence would not require proof. To engage in competition with other men makes a man automatically a part of the problem and not the solution. Caleb is guilty by his own participation in the man to man struggles which have defined him. Had he not identified Falkland as a male other who was first an object of study and then an adversary, he would have avoided his misfortunes; however, his circumstances, things as they are, allowed him only one course.

While it is right, in Godwin's view, to recognize superior characteristics, those characteristics should serve to volitionally and disinterestedly promote human welfare, or happiness, and not to establish a power structure where one man tyrannizes another. "In general terms," as Marilyn Butler has said, "Caleb Williams is about hierarchy,"[73] and, more specifically, the novel demonstrates the inherent evil of social and political structures which pit men against each other and shows how a misinformed belief in the primacy of any one man or any type of male power prevents the realization of societal happiness. Evil occurs when men strive not to unselfishly help each other, but to obtain some advantage over other men.

In Caleb Williams, female characters have limited importance because women were inconsequential to such power relationships in 1794. The masculine old woman who houses the bandits provides the only female threat to male authority when she attempts to kill Caleb. Her appearance and attitude, however, clearly mark her as non-feminine:

> a woman, rather advanced in life, and whose person had I know not what of extraordinary and loathsome. Her eyes were red and blood-shot; her hair was pendant in matted and shaggy tresses about her shoulders; her complexion swarthy, and of the consistency of parchment; her form spare, and her whole body, her arms in particular, uncommonly vigorous and muscular. Not the milk of human kindness, but the feverous blood of savage ferocity, seemed to flow from her heart; and her whole figure suggested an idea of unmitigable energy, and an appetite gorged in malevolence. (249)

Instead of fulfilling a feminine function, the female bandit offers a vitriolic milk, and seems, by her participation in this otherwise male world, to be more perverse and disgusting than any of the men. While Godwin portrays the other female characters in a benevolent manner, they are generally passive victims of the novel's events. For example, Mrs. Jakeman and Mrs. Hammond ineffectual try to save Emily, who, in turn, is unable to save herself. In a sense, Godwin seems to be indicating that females are naturally kinder than males and the unwilling victims of male power struggles; however, when they join in that desire for power, they share (and perhaps exceed) the male propensity for viciousness.

Female characters have so little presence in the novel that we cannot conclude from <u>Caleb Williams</u> much about Godwin's view of the role of women. Their historical exclusion from the institutions and modes of power under scrutiny in the novel precludes any need for Godwin to consider them in depth. The male characters, on the other hand, appear in a variety of forms and expose several conflicting ideological positions which define simultaneously power and manhood. The major male characters, Caleb, Falkland, and Tyrrel, all mistakenly believe that they can become "men" through the acquisition of certain manly characteristics. Caleb seeks knowledge, Falkland privileges honor, and Tyrrel puts his faith in brute force. All fail, however, and their failure demonstrates the futility of their ideologies.

A close reading of <u>Caleb Williams</u> uncovers alternative masculinities, but as Godwin discovered, readers do not always examine a text closely enough to understand its philosophical content. Furthermore, readers share the prejudices of the major male characters when they expect one type of male to overcome the other and consider anything other than a clear victory by one side to be a "curious lack of resolution."[74] Doubts about the reliability of Caleb's narrative voice should make readers question the reliability of the texts they themselves construct, but they are not always inclined to do so. That is part of Godwin's message. "We ought to be upon all occasions prepared to render a reason of our actions,"[75] and we should not assume, like the assumption of the doctrine of optimism, that "whatever is, is right."[76] The perfectibility of man may be possible, but man's errors must first be corrected by an increase in his understanding. At the end of the novel, Caleb's reevaluation of his actions should encourage readers to conduct their own reassessment.

Caleb Williams is not Gothic in the restrictive and pejorative sense which is often associated with that description. Godwin does create a novel of terror, but his terror is Burkean terror, the source of the sublime evoked by contemplating power,[77] and the power Godwin reveals is not supernatural or perverse, but the institutionalized power which men exercise upon each other. Man's mistake is in equating that power with happiness or success. For Godwin, the only route to happiness is in understanding that all power over others is corrupt and corrupting and exists in the companionship found in honest human relationships.

Notes

[1]Thomas De Quincey, Selected Writings of Thomas De Quincey, ed. Philip Van Doren Stern (New York: The Modern Library, 1949) 256-257.

[2]For a full discussion of how the discourse of the eighteenth century used contract terminology to justify patriarchal authority see Carole Pateman, The Sexual Contract (Stanford: Stanford UP, 1988).

[3]William Patrick Day, In the Circles of Fear and Desire (Chicago: U of Chicago P, 1985) 103.

[4]Rudolf F. Storch, "Metaphors of Private Guilt and Social Rebellion in Godwin's Caleb Williams," Journal of English Literary History 34 (1967): 188-207.

[5]Kenneth W. Graham, The Politics of Narrative (New York: AMS P, 1990) 27.

[6]Edith Birkhead, The Tale of Terror (1921; New York: Russell & Russell, 1963) 109.

[7]Peter H. Marshall, William Godwin (New Haven: Yale UP, 1984) 87.

[8]William Godwin, preface, The Adventures of Caleb Williams (New York: Holt, Rinehart & Winston, 1960) xxiii; all subsequent references to Caleb Williams will be made to this edition.

[9]Mark Philp, Godwin's Political Justice (Ithaca: Cornell UP, 1986) 2.

[10]Godwin, preface, CW, xxiii.

[11]Graham, PN, 172.

[12]Godwin, "Godwin's Own Account of Caleb Williams," CW, xxx. These remarks were originally included as part of a preface to Godwin's novel Fleetwood, published in 1832.

[13]Graham, PN, 2

[14]Birkhead 109.

[15]Elizabeth Mac Andrew, The Gothic Tradition in Fiction (New York: Columbia UP, 1979) 96.

[16]Marshall 154.

[17]Marshall 1.

[18]Graham, introduction, PN, 1-10.

[19]Marshall 1.

[20]Kenneth W. Graham, "Gothic Unity," Papers on Language and Literature: A Journal for Scholars and Critics of Language and Literature 20 (1984): 47-59.

[21]Robert Donald Spector, The English Gothic: A Bibliographic Guide to Writers from Horace Walpole to Mary Shelley (Westport, CT: Greenwood P, 1984) 63.

[22]Spector 62.

[23]Everest, Kevin and Gavin Edwards, "William Godwin's Caleb Williams: Truth and 'Things As They Are,' " Reading, Writing, Revolution: Proceedings of the Essex Conference on the Sociology of Literature, July 1981, eds. Francis Barker, et al (Colchester: U of Essex, 1982) 129-146, 131.

[24]Day 83.

[25]Marshall 154.

[26]Marshall 154.

[27]Derek Roper, <u>Reviewing before the Edinburgh, 1788-1802</u> (London: Methuen, 1978) 153.

[28]Graham, <u>PN</u>, 174.

[29]George Sherburn, introduction, <u>Caleb Williams</u>, by William Godwin (New York: Holt, Rinehart & Winston, 1960) viii.

[30]See Graham, <u>PN</u> 175 for mention of Godwin's influence on Southey, Coleridge, and Wordsworth; Graham, <u>PN</u>, 176 (re: Keats); Graham, <u>PN</u>, 177 (re: Byron); and Graham, <u>PN</u>, 180 (re: Shelley).

[31]Graham, <u>PN</u>, 188

[32]D. Gilbert Dumas, "Things as They Were: The Original Ending of <u>Caleb Williams</u>," <u>Studies in English Literature 1500-1900</u> 6 (1966): 575-597.

[33]Graham, "Gothic Unity," 47.

[34]Ken Edward Smith, "William Godwin: social critique in <u>Caleb Williams</u>, <u>Transactions of the Seventh International Congress on the Enlightenment</u>, vol. I (Oxford: The Voltaire Foundation, 1989) 337-341, provides a very brief review of the two sides of this question; Unmentioned by Smith, David McCracken's introduction to his edition of <u>Caleb Williams</u> (London, 1970) vii-xxii, gives a thorough analysis of the connections between <u>Political Justice</u> and <u>Caleb Williams</u> and concludes that Godwin's novel fulfills its political mission; more recently, critics writing in support of the successful connection between the philosophical and the fiction text include Gerald A. Barker, "The Narrative Mode of <u>Caleb Williams</u>: Problems and Resolutions," <u>Studies in the Novel</u> 25 (1993): 1-15; and Kenneth W. Graham, "Narrative and Ideology in Godwin's <u>Caleb Williams</u>," <u>Eighteenth Century Fiction</u> 2 (1990): 215-228; while those who see Godwin's text failing to define his purpose include John Bender, "Impersonal Violence: The Penetrating Gaze and the Field of Narration in <u>Caleb Williams</u>," <u>Critical Reconstructions: The Relationship of Fiction and Life</u>, ed. by Robert M. Polhemus and Roger B. Henkle (Stanford: Stanford UP, 1994) 111-126; and Andrew J. Scheiber, "Falkland's Story: <u>Caleb Williams</u>' Other Voice," <u>Studies in the Novel</u> 17 (1985): 255-266.

[35]Godwin, "Godwin's Own Account," <u>CW</u>, xxv-xxvi.

[36]Karl N. Simms, "Caleb Williams' Godwin: Things as they Are Written," <u>Studies in Romanticism</u> 26 (1987): 343-363.

[37]James Thompson, "Surveillance in William Godwin's <u>Caleb Williams</u>," <u>Gothic Fictions: Prohibition/Transgression</u>, ed. Kenneth W. Graham (New York: AMS P, 1989) 173-198.

[38]Mitzi Myers, "Godwin's Changing Conception of Caleb Williams," <u>Studies in English Literature</u> 12 (1972): 591.

[39]Myers 597.

[40]Myers 624.

[41]Don Locke, <u>A Fantasy of Reason: The Life and Thought of William Godwin</u> (London: Routledge & Kegan Paul, 1980) 73-74.

[42]William Godwin, <u>Enquiry Concerning Political Justice</u>, ed. by K. Codell Carter (Oxford: Clarendon P, 1971) 18.

[43]Philp 108.

[44]Godwin, <u>PJ</u>, 46.

[45]Godwin, <u>PJ</u>, 55.

[46]Godwin, <u>PJ</u>, 183.

[47]Godwin, <u>PJ</u>, 38.

[48]Godwin, <u>PJ</u>, 38.

[49]Godwin, <u>PJ</u>, 171.

[50]Philp 115.

[51]For a summary of this commentary see Graham, "Narrative and Ideology," 217.

[52]Locke 75.

[53]Storch 202.

[54]Locke 73.

[55]Graham, "Narrative and Ideology," 224.

[56]Scheiber 264.

[57]Godwin, <u>PJ</u>, 187.

[58]Godwin, <u>PJ</u>, 188.

[59]Godwin, <u>PJ</u>, 189.

[60]Barker 5.

[61]Storch 201.

[62]Storch 192.

[63]Rajan 240.

[64]McCracken xix.

[65]Marshall 149.

[66]Scheiber 258.

[67]See Godwin, PJ, 188-189.

[68]Wehrs 499.

[69]Michael DePorte, "The Consolations of Fiction: Mystery in Caleb Williams," Papers on Language and Literature: A Journal for Scholars and Critics of Language and Literature 20 (1984) 155.

[70]Bender 121-124.

[71]Philp 111.

[72]Storch 193; see also Myers 604.

[73]Marilyn Butler, "Godwin, Burke, and Caleb Williams," Essays in Criticism 32 (1982): 252.

[74]DePorte 154.

[75]Godwin, PJ, 46.

[76]Alexander Pope, "An Essay on Man," Poetry and Prose of Alexander Pope, ed. by Aubrey Williams (Boston: Houghton Mifflin, 1969) 120-157.

[77]Butler 249.

CHAPTER VIII

CONCLUSION

The man who, in consequence of his unyielding constitution,
cannot fall in with this suppression of instinct, becomes a
"criminal", an "outlaw", in the face of society--unless his social
position or his exceptional capacities enable him to impose
himself upon it as a great man, a 'hero'.

Sigmund Freud[1]

The successful man is an outlaw.

Robert Warshow[2]

My work on male sexuality has only begun. With every page that I
write I discover new questions about how and why man is made in
the image in which he is currently constructed. The villainous male
characters in the Gothic novel appear to represent a resistance to
normal sexuality and have, therefore, given me objects of study
which appear obviously deviant. My intention has been to show how
these deviant sexualities are not so distant from what we recognize
as male sexuality and to explore the complex nature of that sexuality.
The Gothic novel, although only a small part of popular discourse,
provides an example of an alternative genre which, in its historical
presence, seems a symptom for a society in search of a psychosexual
outlet. Because I see the Gothic novel as a symptom, my views on this
genre compare to those of Carol Clover, who in her book about
gender in horror films, <u>Men, Women, and Chain Saws</u>, observes, "To a

remarkable extent, horror has come to seem to me not only the form that most obviously trades in the repressed, but is itself the repressed of mainstream filmmaking."[3] I believe that the labeling of a variety of texts as Gothic has allowed for a too-easily-assumed critical dismissal, and, more importantly, I see the classification of dynamic male characters like Ambrosio, Manfred, Caleb and Falkland on the basis of their abnormality and difference as missing the significance of their sexuality.

Nevertheless, my conclusion to a text about male sexuality and the Gothic novel must necessarily include my own discussion of perversion and power. Unfortunately, this might seem to perpetuate rather than dispel the stereotypes associated with gender and genre studies. In order to clarify the direction of my argument, therefore, I find it important to repeat a basic premise of this thesis: sexuality is diverse, individual, and, henceforth, unclassifiable. The same can be said about novels, especially unique, popular novels which engage the interest of a wide number of people. Studies which attempt to classify and understand the Gothic novel according to the presentation of aberrant sexualities or the aberrant sexualities of its authors presuppose that a normal sexuality, a normal author, and a normal text exist. Studies which ignore and exclude the Gothic novel on the basis of such abnormalities make the same assumption. I believe a more useful approach examines each text for what it represents in terms of defining the boundaries of behavior and the nature of desire. This approach removes the value judgment which is attached to a significant number of widely diverse texts grouped traditionally together as Gothic and calls into question all those constructions which are read as manifestations of masculinity and femininity. Rather than reclassifying or further classifying novels and sexualities, my goal is continually to challenge the classification process.

There is such a thing as the Gothic novel, just as voyeurism, exhibitionism, sadism, masochism, and other perversions do exist. However, both the creation of an alternative genre and the manifestations of alternative sexualities share the need for an authoritative standard from which they can deviate. This standard was seemingly not as apparent to writers in the eighteenth century as it is today, but it was emerging. The attempts to define the woman and the homosexual man at this time were part of this effort to set sexual standards, but an attempt was also being made to define the role of the heterosexual man. Today, it is important to note the failure of this project to restrict female sexuality, to confine women to the home, and to outlaw male homosexuality, but we also need to place a greater importance on the nature and the failure of masculine standards. As I have argued in Chapter Three, the discourse of the eighteenth century increasingly attempts to classify and restrict sexuality, and this structuring of sexuality, in turn, emphasizes a difference between the sexes that presents the woman's body as the unstable and unknowable focus of sexuality in contrast to the unproblematic male body which serves as a consistently ready and willing participant in the sex act. Instead of accepting this oversimplification, we need to question the male body and male sexuality. The widespread existence of male sexual dysfunctions and perverse activity suggests that "normal" masculinity may be just as unreasonable and unrealistic of a standard as the restrictive feminine role which led to the hysterization of women's bodies during the nineteenth century. There is, as Foucault has pointed out, a cause and effect between the powers of societal restraint and the necessary strength of individual resistance, and I see it as no accident that a massively popular genre centered around perverse and aggressive men developed at the same time that the ostensibly benign role of the economic man was being formed.

It is true that the Gothic novel is perverse and about perversion. This should not be read as a pejorative remark, however, because I agree with Robert Stoller that "everyone is perverse"[4] since no one is sexually normal; furthermore, I believe that the Gothic novel, like all perverse activity, occurs as part of a search for a new sexuality which will provide what is missing from the recognized and accepted sexual arrangement. Thus, the rise of the Gothic novel occurs in conjunction with the growing importance of a sexual standard and the inevitable failure of that standard to embody successfully the sexual desires of the individual. The masculinities represented by the Gothic villains suggest alternatives to those suggested by the normative, marriage-bound, young heroes, but these conflicting masculinities share a desire for male power and differ mainly in the means they employ to acquire that power. Manfred and Theodore in Otranto and Ambrosio and Lorenzo in The Monk desire the same things: respectively, the principality of Otranto and the body of Antonia. Perversion is therefore defined in these novels by those characters who clearly do the unacceptable, and the other male characters define normalcy by avoiding such conduct. The problem with these definitions, as I have tried to demonstrate, is that the most active and, hence, masculine males are the villains, who also represent the individual in conflict with society. The popularity of the Gothic novel implies that the deviant sexuality of these men was at least interesting for readers and may suggest that these readers identified with the villains as well as their victims.

The act of reading a critically unacceptable Gothic novel might also suggest that readers were themselves vicariously indulging in perverse behavior when they opened to the pages of one of these disclaimed books. Of course, conclusions regarding the motivations and desires of unknown readers are impossible to make, but given the critical remarks of Wordsworth and Coleridge and Jane Austen's Gothic parody <u>Northanger Abbey</u>, we can assume that readers read the Gothic novel in spite of and often because of its status as an irresponsible genre. The repeated images of symbolic castration found in the often treacherous landscapes, the ruined buildings, and the fragmented bodies may have reflected the growing insecurity of readers in their changing economic (and, consequently, social and political) environment. Austen's novels, for example, display an underlying horror connected to the marriage market which has consequences more real and, therefore, possibly more terrifying than those of the Gothic novel. Significantly, Gothic novels are also marriage narratives, but marriage in these novels is seldom more than a consolation for survival. This formulaic plot resolution follows Gothic chaos, and the reader is returned to a normal world after his or her encounter with the terrifying realm of the Gothic villain. Part of the pleasure of the text is in making this return with those characters who survive and in the reader's recognition that she or he will ultimately escape the castrating forces at work in the text. In other words, the fictionality of the Gothic novel allows the reader to assume a superiority to all the characters, a type of dominance which could be considered similar to that which a voyeur holds over the object of his or her gaze.

In addition to the pleasure readers (from their safe distance) receive from the horror in the text, they may also indulge in the fantasy of a masculinity at war with society as it searches for a completeness which society does not offer or a pleasure which society prohibits. Ambrosio, for example, could accept his monastic responsibilities or leave the church and wander as a vagrant, but these actions would not agree with his and, perhaps, our conception of manhood. Manfred could also cede Otranto at the first sign of confrontation, Falkland and Tyrrel could willingly embrace each other for the sake of social harmony, and Caleb could accept the duties of his lower position in the patriarchal order. These actions would prevent the violence and destruction that these male characters instigate, but this more benign behavior would also reduce them in terms of the phallic power that they associate with manliness. In the end, they display an individual masculinity that conflicts with the role others would prefer them to play, but which more closely aligns itself with its own desire.

Although readers are expected to reject the villain because he goes too far, they do not necessarily reject the power or pleasure he craves. The endings to Otranto and The Monk allow for a transfer of that power to the normative heroes, who receive the principality (power) and the woman (power and pleasure) that the villain sought. In these novels, the issue is not whether males should be in control, but which male should possess that authority. In Caleb Williams, on the other hand, Godwin attempts to show how this emphasis on control of others and hierarchical order destroys everyone; however, because readers still try to assign a winner, either Caleb or Falkland, this point is often overlooked.[5] Readers anticipate that the better man will win and thereby stabilize the novel's conflicting forces, and they desire him to win so that the anxiety created by competing discourses will be alleviated. If, for example, the reader sees either Caleb's economically self-sufficient voice or Falkland's voice of aristocratic values as triumphant at the end of Godwin's novel, then they can close the book with the belief that order has been restored and the values embodied by one of the two characters have been validated. This assumption that things will be set right if the correct man has authority has its roots in patriarchal sovereignty which made legitimacy a question of heredity; however, by the end of the eighteenth century, the question of who should have a legitimate claim to power had come to be discussed in the more difficult terms of conduct. In this effort to define a more correct or more civil behavior for men in authority, however, what was generally examined was the use of power rather than that power itself. Godwin's point appears to be that this desire for power is at the root of human unhappiness; nevertheless, a resistance to ambiguity, or a desire to find a representative which will end insecurity and put things in order, leads even present-day critics to determine the better man in <u>Caleb Williams</u>.

What we struggle with in our attempts to find the best man is our own effort to deny symbolic castration and to locate that symbolic penis which will secure our identities. If we can locate in the aristocratic Falkland or the inventive Caleb those qualities (in the form of signifiers) which will anchor us as men and women through our relationship to those signifiers, then we can more securely traverse a Gothic terrain which threatens our bodily integrity with its images of confinement, emaciation and decay, and physical violence. Symbolically, we can conceal our own lack of being from ourselves by donning the masks of manhood and womanhood and finding appropriate models (in Caleb or Falkland, in this case) with whom we can mirror ourselves. Godwin's message, in my analysis, is that human progress is necessarily connected to a recognition of castration and the taking off of such masks. Such a direction, however, seems impossible as long as we privilege the penis in the establishment of a system which demands gender divisions. This is true whether we divide gender roles into two possibilities (heterosexual), or three or four (with the addition of homosexual roles).

Consequently, as the Oedipus complex continues to supply us with what we have interpreted as these gendered identities, male heterosexuality continues to be associated with a power which females and male homosexuals both protest and try to equal. We cannot argue for equal power among gendered individuals without simultaneously supporting those differences which assign gender. Alan Bray's excellent study of the emergence of the homosexual community shows how Enlightenment ideology with its analytic processes and focus on the particular categorized and condemned simultaneously as it segregated and thus made male homosexuality consequential.[6] Bray has shown how the same ideological factors which try to label and exclude also aggrandize their subjects by assigning them a previously undiscussed significance, albeit a highly negative one. This process also works in reverse with increased significance causing more apparent difference. In addition, this creation of the homosexual as a third or fourth gender,[7] demonstrates how the Oedipus complex has served as the dividing line among those who would identify with the mother or father and how the penis functions as the difference between those expected identifications. Randolph Trumbach's research[8] supports Freud's observation that female homosexuality had "been ignored by the law,"[9] at least, apparently, through the nineteenth century. This lack of concern with female homosexuality exemplifies a civilization more apprehensive of the nature of male subjectivity, or how men come to be identified in relation to the symbolic penis of the father. If males deny the father or assume the mother's feminine role in his seduction, they imply a kind of lawlessness which refuses to acknowledge the superior power of the penis that the patriarchy grants to males. In effect, male homosexuality must be outlawed if male heterosexuality is to have social value.

The institutionalization of a process which classifies males according to their sexual relationship with other males can be seen as coexistent with the tightening of restraints on male homosexuality; however, it can also be seen as part of the larger attempt to restrict male sexuality and to limit the functions and pleasures of the male body. If life for men desiring homosexual relationships changed at this time, it can be presumed that the nature of male heterosexual relationships was also altered. An increasing amount of social and legal discourse and action intervened in the sexual lives of individuals and privileged and prohibited certain behaviors. The male sexual hierarchy, like the social hierarchy, began to have its outcasts (traditionally, homosexuals), its lower class (certain perverts), its middle class (the undiscussed "normal" male) and its upper class (men of power and pleasure). With this growing emphasis on sexual restraint, one result for males was a sublimation of sexual desire into production and an increasing identification with one's labor around this time. In his book on the gender changes which take place in the 300 years prior to the nineteenth century, Anthony Fletcher describes an emerging "masculine honour code"[10] which "prescribed soberness, authority, [as well as] steady and honest labour," all qualities which related to a more civil and polite male behavior that simultaneously retained control over females while encouraging commerce among men. The growing importance of these qualities during the eighteenth century has an importance today because of their resemblance to the characteristics typically included in the modern male sex role[11] which social scientists point to as the standard of manhood with which the majority of males identify.

A discussion of the problems surrounding male sexuality should begin with this traditional masculine role and not be limited to those individuals considered physically or psychologically diseased, deformed, or otherwise different. Feminists have demonstrated that sexuality has historically been associated with power relations, and male sexuality, in particular, has been linked to a control and power over others. In this text, I have tried to show how the Gothic villain, in spite of his clearly anti-social nature, exhibits a sexuality that we equate with a powerful masculinity. To a less obvious extent, however, the majority of male sexualities currently relate to the same phallic power source. Although few men have the seemingly limitless access to pleasure of a Gothic villain or a Hollywood star, they usually acquire something (a material possession, a career, a woman, etc.) which will provide a masculine identification. The desire for males to prove themselves in a multitude of various ways needs further study, and this study should question male roles regardless of their social acceptability.

Like the surviving normative characters in a Gothic novel, we might all rest easier if the Gothic villain, as the representative of an anti-societal and often violent masculinity, were truly dead. However, the symbolic power of this villain lives on not only in his obvious descendants such as Jason (<u>Friday the 13th</u>), Freddy (<u>Nightmare on Elm Street</u>), Michael (<u>Halloween</u>) and other "slasher" males, but also in those representations of masculinity characterized by action heroes, Godfather-type villain-heroes, or ruthless business-men whose type was portrayed by Michael Douglas in the movie <u>Wall Street</u>. While slasher villains continue the Gothic tradition established in <u>Otranto</u> of showing a sexually-troubled male in pursuit of beautiful, young females, the men in these other films are preoccu-pied with defining themselves in terms of power, perhaps more in the manner of <u>Caleb Williams</u>. Typically, this means that men whom the audience is cued to identify as good are pitted against those whom the audience identifies as bad. In the action movie, the bad men often commit or threaten to commit a heinous crime which results or promises to result in the deaths of hundreds, thousands, or millions, and this provides the hero with the opportunity to do his own share of killing in defense of all those innocent lives which are endangered. These opposing types of men, consequently, exhibit similar behavior which differs only in respect to motive. In True Lies, when the character played by Jamie Lee Curtis asks Arnold Schwarzenegger's heroic character if he has killed a lot of men, he replies, "Yes, but they were all bad."[12] The humor intended for this line relies on the audience's recognition of the obviously fictional nature of the action genre and the clear distinction which occurs between good and bad, a distinction not easily made in real life. In films which focus more subtly on criminal behavior, such distinctions are generally blurred and the hero can be Don Corleone, a man whose ruthlessness leads him to power in The Godfather, or a combination of criminal and police detective, like in the movie Heat, where characters played by Robert DeNiro and Al Pacino are shown as mirror images of each other on opposing sides of the law.

This appropriation of the mirror image, or doppelganger, to show difference and resemblance is also a common occurrence in the Gothic. For example, Caleb Williams and Falkland can be seen as doubles,[13] and, in the course of the novel, each man forms his identity in relation to the other. In the end, when Falkland dies, Caleb has "no character"[14] left and is, in effect, without an identity because the other which defined him is gone. Like Heat's policeman/criminal opposition, Falkland and Caleb seemingly force the other to take destructive action and exist only in symbolic difference to each other. Because the law differentiates the two men, they establish a relationship which depends entirely on their symbolic meaning and loses all connection to the realities of their body, their lived experience. Our

241

study of male sexuality needs to go beyond a study of the two sides of the doppelganger and to explore the body which both constructions avoid. We need to begin by questioning the key assumptions of the nature of human sexuality and its relationship to both the body and the power which society recognizes in the performance of certain sex roles.

Historian Fletcher has said that the "simple fact is that men revised a scheme of gender relations that served their interests as men so effectively during the three centuries from 1500 to 1800 that it has survived."[15] While I do not question that heterosexual men obtained a type of limited power over the other gender(s) which generally harmed those genders during this time, I believe it is wrong to imagine that this scheme of gender relations worked effectively to the interests of the majority of males. Such a conclusion assumes that this type of sexual power provides the greatest possible pleasure, and, by making this assumption, pays homage to the phallic authority of the mythical primal father (who had unrestricted access to sexual pleasure). This conclusion also fails to acknowledge those men whose lives seem by no means enriched by their male authority. What of the countless numbers of men who have died in battle, who have failed to achieve dominion over property (real, personal, or female), or who have, in spite or because of their accomplishments, always felt incomplete, anxious, or guilty? Rather than locating a winner in this battle of the genders, I see both males and females detrimentally harmed by the roles they have been assigned. In my revisioning of gender roles, I hope to promote that which has too often been left out of gender studies: the pleasures found in the absolute difference of each individual and the power of that relinquishment of self which accompanies an abandonment of materialistic values and that ideal relationship between beings which can only be termed love.

In writing a dissertation on male subjectivity, I have used terms like "male", "masculine", and "man" so often that I have come to question whether any of them has a fixed meaning. Perhaps that is my ultimate point. Certainly Freud saw these terms as meaningless to the newborn child. We are, after all, each uniquely sexual and our interpretations of our world are based upon that sexuality, which spans the active and passive, the masculine and feminine.[16] It is our understanding of this sexual uniqueness which should lead us to suspect all attempts to classify gender. Furthermore, we need to recognize our own mortality as well as the mortality of others. If we can come to embrace our inevitable incompleteness and to care for others because they share that lack of totality that each of us psychically experiences, then perhaps we can begin to learn a new type of power unpredicated on the mythical father's omnipotence. Kaja Silverman, in her most recent book, has suggested that we begin to reimage ourselves with an understanding of our own imperfectability, or that we look at others and ourselves as "good enough," rather than attempting to locate the perfect image.[17] Her analysis includes the observation that an active idealization of these less than perfect images of the other and the active gift of love for that other would cause "reverberations" that could "resound within the entire field of a given subject's interpersonal relations."[18] My suggestion is that our relationship to the other's body is always one of desire, even when that desire is experienced as fear or revulsion. When we are able to recognize that we truly desire both the mother's and the father's love in all of their many manifestations in the field of the other, then the competition which renders the Oedipus complex in its current form will be transformed into a more ethical use of energy.

For the male body, a recognition of insufficiency is an uncharacteristic and, therefore, difficult but important first step. The penis, so long prized and privileged, needs to be devalued and "de-meaned." Released from the "tyranny" of the penis,[19] males might begin to find sexual pleasure in an increasing number of ways with their whole body. Unconcerned with the demands of compulsory heterosexuality, perhaps they can enjoy both the biological difference of females and the biological similarity of other males in ways that resemble a mutuality more than a competition or a will to power. However, the narcissistic fantasy of completion is an alluring one, and the pride the male takes in his biological signification (his penis) is supported by a preponderance of cultural stigmata. If he has any hope of escaping the gender role that currently imprisons him, he must explore the sexual nature of the other regions of his body, and he must begin to see the other as his equally imperfect equal.

Notes

[1]Sigmund Freud, " 'Civilized' Sexual Morality and Modern Nervous Illness," Freud on Women: A Reader, ed. Elisabeth Young-Bruehl (New York: Norton, 1990) 167.

[2]Robert Warshow, "The Gangster as Tragic Hero," Reading Culture, eds. Diana George and John Trimbur, 2nd ed. (New York: HarperCollins, 1995) 377.

[3]Carol J. Clover, Men, Women, and Chain Saws: Gender in the Modern Horror Film (Princeton: Princeton UP, 1992) 20.

[4]Robert Stoller, "The Term Perversion," Perversions and Near-Perversions in Clinical Practice: New Psychoanalytic Perspectives, eds. Gerald I. Fogel and Wayne A. Myers (New Haven: Yale UP, 1991) 53.

[5]See Chapter Seven, 216; for two differing views on who "wins" the Caleb/Falkland struggle, see Mitzi Myers, "Godwin's Changing Conception of Caleb Williams," Studies in English Literature 12 (1972) 591, and Don Locke, A Fantasy of Reason: The Life and Thought of William Godwin (London: Routledge & Kegan Paul, 1980) 73-74.

[6]Alan Bray, Homosexuality in Renaissance England (London: Gay Men's Press, 1982).

[7]See Randolph Trumbach, "The Birth of the Queen: Sodomy and the Emergence of Gender Equality in Modern Culture, 1660-1750," Hidden

From History: Reclaiming the Gay and Lesbian Past, eds. Martin Bauml Duberman et al. (New York: NAL Books, 1989) 129-140.

[8]Randolph Trumbach, "London's Sodomites: Homosexual Behavior and Western Culture in Eighteenth Century, Journal of Social History 11 (1977) 13.

[9]Sigmund Freud, "The Psychogenesis of a Case of Homosexuality in a Woman," Freud on Women: A Reader, ed. Elisabeth Young-Bruehl (New York: Norton, 1990) 242.

[10]Anthony Fletcher, Gender, Sex and Subodination in England 1500-1800 (New Haven: Yale UP, 1995) 402.

[11]See the Introduction, 5; See also R. W. Connell, Gender and Power: Society, the Person and Sexual Politics (Stanford: Stanford UP, 1987) 183; David D. Gilmore, Manhood in the Making: Cultural Concepts of Masculinity (New Haven: Yale UP, 1990) 10; and Joseph H. Pleck, The Myth of Masculinity (Cambridge: MIT P, 1981) 140-141.

[12]James Cameron, director, True Lies, perf. Arnold Schwarzenegger and Jamie Lee Curtis, Twentieth Century Fox, 1994.

[13]William Patrick Day, In the Circles of Fear and Desire (Chicago: U of Chicago P, 1985) 137.

[14]William Godwin, Caleb Williams or Things as They Are (New York: Holt, Rinehart & Winston, 1965) 378.

[15]Fletcher 430.

[16]Sigmund Freud, "Some Psychical Consequences of the Anatomical Distinction Between the Sexes," Freud on Women: A Reader, ed. Elisabeth Young-Bruehl (New York: Norton, 1990) 307.

[17]Kaja Silverman, The Threshold of the Visible World (New York: Routledge, 1996).

[18]Silverman 80.

[19]See my comments on the greater tyranny of the penis in Chapter One, 35-36.

Works Cited

Amussen, Susan Dwyer. <u>An Ordered Society: Gender and Class in Early Modern England</u>. Oxford: Basil Blackwell, 1988.

Anderson, Howard. "Gothic Heroes." <u>The English Hero, 1660-1800</u>. Ed. Robert Folkenflik. Newark: U of Delaware P, 1982. 205-221.

Armstrong, Nancy. <u>Desire and Domestic Fiction.</u> New York: Oxford UP, 1987.

Armstrong, Nancy and Leonard Tennenhouse. <u>The Imaginary Puritan: Literature, Intellectual Labor, and the Origins of Personal Life</u>. Berkeley: U of California P, 1992.

Austen, Jane. <u>Northanger Abbey, Persuasion, Emma.</u> Leicester: Galley, 1988.

Bakhtin, Mikhail. <u>The Dialogic Imagination</u>. Ed. Michael Holquist. Trans. Caryyl Emerson and Michael Holquist. Austin: U of Texas P, 1981.

Baldridge, Cates. <u>The Dialogics of Dissent in the English Novel.</u> Hanover, NH: Middlebury College P, 1994.

Ballaster, Ros. <u>Seductive Forms: Women's Amatory Fiction from 1684 to 1740</u>. Oxford: Clarendon P, 1992.

Barker, Gerald A. "The Narrative Mode of <u>Caleb Williams</u>: Problems and Resolutions." <u>Studies in the Novel</u> 25 (1993): 1-15.

Barthes, Roland. <u>Sade/ Fourier/ Loyola.</u> Trans. Richard Miller. Berkeley: U of California P, 1989.

Bayer-Berenbaum, Linda. <u>The Gothic Imagination.</u> Rutherford: Fairleigh Dickinson UP, 1982.

Begg, Ean. "Animus: the Unmentionable Archetype." <u>Choirs of the God: Revisioning Masculinity</u>. Ed. John Matthews. London: Mandala, 1991. 151-168.

Behrendt, Stephen C. "Questioning the Romantic Novel." <u>Studies in the Novel</u> 26.2 (1994): 5-25.

Bender, John. "Impersonal Violence: The Penetrating Gaze and the Field of Narration in <u>Caleb Williams</u>." <u>Critical Reconstructions: The Relationship of Fiction and Life</u>. Ed. Robert M. Polhemus and Roger B. Henkle. Stanford: Stanford UP, 1994. 111-126.

Bernbaum, Ernest. <u>Guide through the Romantic Movement</u>. New York: Ronald P, 1930.

Bernstein, Stephen. "Form and Ideology in the Gothic Novel." <u>Essays in Literature</u> 18 (1991): 151-165.

Berryman, John. Introduction. <u>The Monk</u>. By Matthew G. Lewis. New York: Grove P, 1952. 11-28.

Birkhead, Edith. <u>The Tale of Terror: A Study of the Gothic Romance</u>. London: Constable, 1921.

Bloch, Ruth H. "Untangling the Roots of Modern Sex Roles: A Survey of Four Centuries of Change." <u>Signs</u> 4 (1978): 237-252.

Bracher, Mark. <u>Lacan, Discourse, and Social Change: A Psychoanalytic Cultural Criticism</u>. Ithaca: Cornell UP, 1993.

Bray, Alan. <u>Homosexuality in Renaissance England.</u> London: Gay Men's Press, 1982.

Brenkman, John. <u>Straight Male Modern: A Cultural Critique of Psychoanalysis</u>. New York: Routledge, 1993.

Brod, Harry. "A Case for Men's Studies." <u>Changing Men: New Directions in Research on Men and Masculinity</u>. Ed. Michael Kimmel. Newbury Park: Sage, 1987.

Brooks, Peter. "Virtue and Terror: <u>The Monk</u>," <u>ELH</u> 40 (1973): 249-263.

Bly, Robert. <u>Iron John.</u> Reading, MA: Addison-Wesley, 1990.

---. "The Hawk, the Horse and the Rider." <u>Choirs of the God: Revisioning Masculinity</u>. Ed. John Matthews. London: Mandala, 1991. 13-28.

Breitenburg, Mark. <u>Anxious Masculinity in Early Modern England</u>. Cambridge: Cambridge UP, 1996.

Brod, Harry. "A Case for Men's Studies." <u>Changing Men: New Directions in Research on Men and Masculinity</u>. Ed. Michael Kimmel. Newbury Park: Sage, 1987. 263-277.

Bueler, Lois E. <u>Clarissa's Plots.</u> Newark: U of Del P, 1994.

Burke, Edmund. <u>Reflections on the Revolution in France</u>. Ed. Thomas H. D. Mahoney. New York: Macmillan, 1955.

Burney, Fanny. <u>Evelina or, A Young Lady's Entrance into the World</u>. London: Dent, 1958.

Butler, Marilyn. "Godwin, Burke, and <u>Caleb Williams</u>." <u>Essays in Criticism</u> 32 (1982): 237-257.

Castle, Terry. "The Spectralization of the Other in <u>The Mysteries of Udolpho</u>." <u>The New Eighteenth Century</u>. Ed. Felicity Nussbaum and Laura Brown. New York: Methuen, 1989. 231-253.

Chodorow, Nancy. <u>The Reproduction of Mothering</u>. Berkeley: U of California P, 1978.

Clatterbaugh, Kenneth. <u>Contemporary Perspectives on Masculinity.</u> Boulder: Westview P, 1990.

Cleland, John. <u>Memoirs of a Woman of Pleasure</u> or <u>Fanny Hill</u>. Hertfordshire: Wordsworth Editions, 1993.

Clover, Carol J. <u>Men, Women, and Chain Saws: Gender in the Modern Horror Film</u>. Princeton: Princeton UP, 1992.

Coleridge, Samuel Taylor. <u>The Table Talk and Omniana of Samuel Taylor Coleridge</u>. London: Humphrey Milford: Oxford UP, 1917.

Conger, Syndy M. "Sensibility Restored: Radcliffe's Answer to Lewis's <u>The Monk</u>." <u>Gothic Fictions: Prohibition/Transgression</u>. Ed. Kenneth W. Graham. New York: AMS P, 1989. 113-149.

Connell, R. W. <u>Gender and Power: Society, the Person and Sexual Politics</u>. Stanford: Stanford UP, 1987.

Corneau, Guy. <u>Absent Fathers, Lost Sons: The Search for Masculine Identity.</u> Trans. Larry Shouldice. Boston: Shambala, 1991.

Crisp, Quentin. Introduction. <u>Quentin Crisp's Book of Quotations: 1000 Observations on Life and Love by, for, and about Gay Men and Women.</u> New York: Macmillan, 1989.

Day, William Patrick. <u>In the Circles of Fear and Desire.</u> Chicago: U of Chicago P, 1985.

DePorte, Michael. "The Consolations of Fiction: Mystery in Caleb Williams." <u>Papers on Language and Literature: A Journal for Scholars and Critics of Language and Literature</u> 20 (1984): 154-164.

De Quincey, Thomas. <u>Selected Writings of Thomas De Quincey.</u> Ed. Philip Van Doren Stern. New York: The Modern Library, 1949.

Deutsch, Helene. "The Psychology of Women in Relation to the Functions of Reproduction (1924)." <u>Women & Analysis: Dialogues on Psychoanalytic Views of Femininity.</u> Ed. Jean Strouse. Boston: G. K. Hall, 1985. 147-161.

Doody, Margaret Anne. <u>A Natural Passion: A Study of the Novels of Samuel Richardson.</u> Oxford: Clarendon P, 1974.

Dumas, D. Gilbert. "Things as They Were: The Original Ending of <u>Caleb Williams</u>." <u>Studies in English Literature 1500-1900</u> 6 (1966): 575-597.

Eagleton, Terry. <u>The Rape of Clarissa</u>. Minneapolis: U of Minn P, 1982.

Easthope, Antony. <u>What a Man's Gotta Do: The Masculine Myth in Popular Culture</u>. Boston: Unwin Hyman, 1986.

Elliot, Patricia. <u>From Mastery to Analysis: Theories of Gender inPsychoanalytic Feminism</u>. Ithaca: Cornell UP, 1991.

Ellis, Kate Ferguson. <u>The Contested Castle: Gothic Novels and the Subversion of Domestic Ideology.</u> Urbana: U of Illinois P, 1989.

Everest, Kevin and Gavin Edwards. "William Godwin's <u>Caleb Williams</u>: Truth and 'Things As They Are.' " <u>Reading, Writing, Revolution: Proceedings of the Essex Conference on the Sociology of Literature</u>, July 1981. Eds. Francis Barker, et al. Colchester: U of Essex, 1982. 129-146.

Faludi, Susan. <u>Backlash: The Undeclared War Against Women.</u> London: Vintage, 1992.

Farrell, Warren. The Liberated Man. New York: Bantam, 1974.

Fielding, Henry. Joseph Andrews and Shamela. London: Oxford UP, 1971.

---. Tom Jones. New York: New American Library, 1963.

Foucault, Michel. The History of Sexuality. Trans. Robert Hurley. New York: Pantheon, 1978.

---. The Use of Pleasure. Trans. Robert Hurley. New York: Pantheon, 1985.

Frank, Frederick S. Introduction. Gothic Fiction: A Master List of Twentieth Century Criticism and Research. Westport: Meckler, 1988. ix-xiv.

---. Preface. The First Gothics: A Critical Guide to the English Gothic Novel. New York: Garland, 1987. ix-xxx.

---. "The Gothic Romance 1762-1820." Horror Literature. Ed. M. B. Tymn. New York: Bowker, 1981. 3-33.

Franklin, Clyde W. The Changing Definition of Masculinity. New York: Plenum P, 1984.

Freud, Sigmund. A Case of Hysteria, Three Essays on Sexuality and Other Works. Vol VII of The Complete Psychological Works. London: Hogarth, 1953, 1981.

---. " 'Civilized' Sexual Morality and Modern Nervous Illness." Freud on Women: A Reader. Ed. Elisabeth Young-Bruehl. New York: Norton, 1990. 166-181.

---. "The Psychogenesis of a Case of Homosexuality in a Woman." Freud on Women: A Reader. Ed. Elisabeth Young-Bruehl. New York: Norton, 1990. 241-266.

---. Totem and Taboo and Other Works. Vol XIII of The Complete Psychological Works. London: Hogarth, 1955, 1981.

Frye, Northrup. Anatomy of Criticism: Four Essays. Princeton: Princeton UP, 1957.

Gallagher, Catherine. Nobody's Story: The Vanishing Acts of Women Writers in the Marketplace 1670-1820. Berkeley: U of Cal P, 1994.

Gallop, Jane. Around 1981: Academic Feminist Literary Theory. New York: Routledge, 1992.

Geary, Robert. The Supernatural in Gothic Fiction. Lewiston: Edward Mellen P, 1992.

Gilmore, David D. Manhood in the Making: Cultural Concepts of Masculinity. New Haven: Yale UP, 1990.

Godwin, William. Caleb Williams or Things as They Are. New York: Holt, Rinehart & Winston, 1965.

---. Enquiry Concerning Political Justice. Ed. K. Codell Carter. Oxford: Clarendon P, 1971.

---. "Godwin's Own Account of Caleb Williams." Caleb Williams. By Godwin. New York: Holt, Rinehart & Winston, 1960. xxv-xxx.

---. Preface. Caleb Williams. By Godwin. New York: Holt, Rinehart & Winston, 1960. xxiii-xxiv.

---. The Enquirer: Reflections on Education, Manners and Literature. New York: August M. Kelley, 1965.

Graham, Kenneth W. "Afterword: Some Remarks on Gothic Origins." Gothic Fictions: Prohibition/Transgression. New York: AMS P, 1989. 259 - 268.

---. "Gothic Unity." Papers on Language and Literature: A Journal for Scholars and Critics of Language and Literature 20 (1984): 47-59.

---. "Narrative and Ideology in Godwin's Caleb Williams." Eighteenth Century Fiction 2 (1990): 215-228.

---. The Politics of Narrative. New York: AMS P, 1990.

Green, Katherine Sobba. The Courtship Novel, 1740-1820: A Feminized Genre. Lexington: UP of Kentucky, 1991.

Greveson, Jonathan. "Health or Home." Men, Sex and Relationships. Ed. Victor J. Seidler. London: Routledge, 1992. 111-113.

Gwilliam, Tassie. Samuel Richardson's Fictions of Gender. Stanford: Stanford UP, 1993.

Haggerty, George. "Literature and Homosexuality in the Late Eighteenth Century: Walpole, Beckford, and Lewis." Studies in the Novel 18 (1986): 341-352.

---. "The Gothic Novel, 1764-1824," The Columbia History of the British Novel. Ed. John Richetti. New York: Columbia UP, 1994. 220-246.

Hall, Leslie. Hidden Anxieties. Cambridge: Polity P, 1991.

Harfst, Betsy Perteit. Horace Walpole and the Unconscious: an Experiment in Freudian Analysis. New York: Arno Press, 1980.

Harris, Jocelyn. Introduction. The History of Sir Charles Grandison. Vol. I. By Samuel Richardson. London: Oxford, 1972. vii-xxiv.

Herek, Gregory M. "Reformulating the Male Role." Changing Men: New Directions in Research on Men and Masculinity. Ed. Michael Kimmel. Newbury Park: Sage, 1987. 71-76.

Hill, Christopher. Some Intellectual Consequences of the English Revolution. Madison: U of Wisconsin P, 1980.

Horney, Karen. "The Flight from Womanhood: The Masculinity-Complex in Women as Viewed by Men and by Women (1926)." Women & Analysis: Dialogues on Psychoanalytic Views of Femininity. Ed. Jean Strouse. Boston: G. K. Hall, 1985. 171-186.

Howard, Jacqueline. Reading Gothic Fiction: A Bakhtinian Approach. Oxford: Clarendon P, 1994.

Hume, Robert D. "Gothic Versus Romantic: A Revaluation of the Gothic Novel." PMLA 84 (1969): 282-290.

Irigaray, Luce. This Sex Which is Not One. Trans. Catherine Porter. Ithaca: Cornell UP, 1977, 1985.

Jones, Chris. Radical Sensibility: Literature and Ideas in the 1790s. London: Routledge, 1993

Kallich, Martin. Horace Walpole. New York: Twayne, 1971.

Kestenberg, Judith. "Outside and Inside, Male and Female." The Journal of the American Psychoanalytic Association 16 (1968): 457-520.

Keymer, Tom. "Clarissa's Death, Clarissa's Sale, and the Text of the Second Edition," The Review of English Studies 45 (1994): 388-396.

---. Richardson's Clarissa and the Eighteenth-Century Reader. Cambridge: Cambridge UP, 1992.

Kimmel, Michael. "Teaching a Course on Men: Masculinist Reaction or 'Gentlemen's Auxiliary'?" <u>Changing Men: New Directions in Research on Men and Masculinity</u>. Ed. Kimmel. Newbury Park: Sage, 1987. 278-294.

Kraft, Elizabeth. "Public Nurturance and Private Civility: The Transposition of Values in Eighteenth-Century Fiction." <u>Studies in Eighteenth-Century Culture</u>. Eds. Patricia B. Craddock and Carla H. Hay. Vol. 22. East Lansing, MI: Colleagues P, 1992. 181-193.

Lacan, Jacques. <u>Ecrits.</u> Trans. Alan Sheridan. New York: Norton, 1977.

---. <u>Feminine Sexuality</u>. Trans. Jacqueline Rose. Ed. Juliet Mitchell and Jacqueline Rose. New York: Norton, 1982.

---. <u>The Four Fundamental Concepts of Psycho-Analysis</u>. Trans. Alan Sheridan. New York: Norton, 1981.

Lamont, Claire. "The Romantic Period: 1780-1830." <u>An Outline of English Literature</u>. Ed. Pat Rogers. Oxford: Oxford UP, 1992. 250-298.

Laqueur, Thomas. <u>Making Sex: Body and Gender from the Greeks to Freud</u>. Cambridge, MA: Harvard UP, 1990.

Le Tellier, R. I. <u>An Intensifying Vision of Evil: The Gothic Novel (1764 - 1820) as a Self-Contained Literary Cycle</u>. Salzburg: Universitat Salzburg, 1980.

---. <u>Kindred Spirits: Interrelations and Affinities between the Romantic Novels of England and Germany (1790-1820).</u> Salzburg: Universitat Salzburg, 1982.

Lee, Jonathan Scott. <u>Jacques Lacan</u>. Amherst: U of Massachusetts P, 1990.

Lewis, Matthew G. <u>The Monk.</u> New York: Grove Press, 1952.

Lewis, Wilmarth Sheldon. <u>Horace Walpole</u>. New York: Pantheon Books, 1960.

Locke, Don. <u>A Fantasy of Reason: The Life and Thought of William Godwin</u>. London: Routledge & Kegan Paul, 1980.

Locke, John. <u>Of Civil Government, Second Treatise</u>. Chicago: Gateway, 1955.

Mac Andrew, Elizabeth. The Gothic Tradition in Fiction. New York: Columbia UP, 1979.

Mackensie, Henry. The Man of Feeling. London: Oxford UP, 1967.

Magistrale, Tony. "More Demon than Man: Melville's Ahab as Gothic Villain." Spectrum of the Fantastic. Ed. Donald Palumbo. Westport, CT: Greenwood, 1988. 81 - 86.

Markley, Robert. Fallen Languages. Ithaca: Cornell UP, 1993.

Marks, Sylvia Kasey. Sir Charles Grandison: The Compleat Conduct Book. Lewisburg: Bucknell UP, 1986.

Marshall, Peter H. William Godwin. New Haven: Yale UP, 1984.

Matthews, John. Introduction. Choirs of the God: Revisioning Masculinity. Ed. Matthews. London: Mandala, 1991. 9-12.

---. Notes on Contributors. Choir of the God: Revisioning Masculinity. Ed. Matthews. London: Mandala, 1991. 215-217.

Mayo, Robert D. The English Novel in the Magazines 1740-1815. Evanston: Northwestern UP, 1962.

Mazlish, Bruce. Kissinger: The European Mind in American Policy. New York: Basic Books, 1976.

McCracken, David. Introduction. Caleb Williams. By William Godwin. London: Oxford UP, 1970. vii-xxii.

McKeon, Michael. "Historicizing Patriarchy: The Emergence of Gender Difference in England, 1660-1760." Eighteenth-Century Studies 28 (1995): 295-322.

Mehrotra, K. K. Horace Walpole and the English Novel: A Study of the Influence of "The Castle of Otranto" 1764-1820. New York: Russell & Russell, 1934, 1970.

Miles, Rosalind. Love, Sex, Death, and the Making of the Male. New York: Summit, 1991.

Millett, Kate. Sexual Politics. New York: Doubleday, 1970.

Mitchell, Juliet. Introduction-I. Feminine Sexuality: Jacques Lacan and the "école freudienne". Ed. Mitchell and Jacqueline Rose. New York: Norton, 1982. 1-26.

---. "On Freud and the Distinction Between the Sexes." Women & Analysis: Dialogues on Psychoanalytic Views of Femininity. Ed. Jean Strouse. Boston: G. K. Hall, 1985. 27-36.

---. Psycho-Analysis and Feminism. New York: Vintage, 1974.

Money, John. Gay, Straight, and In-Between: The Sexology of Erotic Orientation. New York: Oxford UP, 1988.

Moore, Robert and Douglas Gillette. The Magician Within: Accessing the Shaman in the Male Psyche. New York: William Morrow, 1993.

Myers, Mitzi. "Godwin's Changing Conception of Caleb Williams." Studies in English Literature 12 (1972): 591-628.

Nicholson, Linda J. Gender and History: The Limits of Social Theory in the Age of the Family. New York: Columbia UP, 1986.

Nussbaum, Felicity and Laura Brown, eds. The New Eighteenth Century. New York: Methuen, 1989.

Parreaux, André. The Publication of "The Monk": A Literary Event 1796-1798. Paris: Didier, 1960.

Pateman, Carole. The Sexual Contract. Stanford: Stanford UP, 1988.

Peck, Louis F. A Life of Matthew G. Lewis. Cambridge: Harvard UP, 1961.

Philp, Mark. Godwin's Political Justice. Ithaca: Cornell UP, 1986.

Pleck, Joseph H. The Myth of Masculinity. Cambridge: MIT P, 1981.

Plummer, Ken. "Sexual Diversity: A Sociological Perspective." The Psychology of Sexual Diversity. Ed Kevin Howells. Oxford: Basil Blackwell, 1984. 219-253.

Pope, Alexander. "An Essay on Man." Poetry and Prose of Alexander Pope. Ed. Aubrey Williams. Boston: Houghton Mifflin, 1969. 120-157.

Porter, Roy. "Mixed Feelings: the Enlightenment and Sexuality in Eighteenth-Century Britain." Sexuality in Eighteenth-Century Britain. Ed. Paul-Gabriel Boucé. Manchester: Manchester UP, 1982. 1-27.

Price, John Valdimir. "Patterns of Sexual Behavior in Some Eighteenth-Century Novels." <u>The Country Myth</u>. Ed. H. George Hahn. Frankfurt: Peter Lang, 1990. 125-138.

Probyn, Clive. <u>English Fiction of the Eighteenth Century</u>. London: Longman, 1987.

Punter, David. <u>The Literature of Terror: A History of Gothic Fictions from 1765 to the Present Day</u>. London: Longman, 1980.

---. "Narrative and Psychology in Gothic Fiction." <u>Gothic Fictions: Prohibition/Transgression</u>. Ed. Kenneth W. Graham. New York: AMS P, 1989. 1-28.

Radcliffe, Ann. <u>The Italian or Confessional of the Black Penitants</u>. London: Oxford UP, 1968.

---. <u>The Mysteries of Udolpho.</u> London: Dent, 1931.

Ragland-Sullivan, Ellie. "The Sexual Masquerade: A Lacanian Theory of Sexual Difference." <u>Lacan and the Subject of Language</u>. Ed. Ragland-Sullivan and Mark Bracher. New York: Routledge, 1991. 49-80.

Railo, Eino. <u>The Haunted Castle: A Study of the Elements of English Romanticism</u>. London: Routledge, 1927.

Richardson, Samuel. <u>Clarissa.</u> 4 vols. London: Dent, 1985.

---. <u>The History of Sir Charles Grandison</u>. Ed. Jocelyn Harris. Vol. I. London: Oxford, 1972.

---. <u>Pamela.</u> New York: Viking Penguin, 1980.

Roper, Derek. <u>Reviewing before the Edinburgh, 1788-1802</u>. London: Methuen, 1978.

Roper, Lyndal. <u>Oedipus and the Devil: Witchcraft, Sexuality and Religion in Early Modern Europe</u>. London: Routledge, 1994.

Rose, Jacqueline. Introduction-II. <u>Feminine Sexuality: Jacques Lacan and the "école freudienne"</u>. Ed. Juliet Mitchell and Rose. New York: Norton, 1982. 27-57.

Rosen, David. <u>The Changing Fictions of Masculinity</u>. Urbana: U of Illinois P, 1993.

Rowan, John. The Horned God. London: Routledge, 1987.

Scheiber, Andrew J. "Falkland's Story: Caleb Williams' Other Voice." Studies in the Novel 17 (1985): 255-266.

Schellenberg, Betty A. "Using 'Femalities' to 'Make Fine Men': Richardson's Sir Charles Grandison and the Feminization of Narrative." Studies in English Literature, 1500-1800 34 (1994): 599-616.

Sedgwick, Eve Kosofsky. Between Men. New York: Columbia UP, 1985.

---. "The Character in the Veil: Imagery of the Surface in the Gothic Novel," PMLA 96 (1981): 255-270.

---. The Coherence of Gothic Conventions. New York: Methuen, 1986.

Seidler, Victor. "Men, Sex and Relationships." Men, Sex and Relationships. Ed. Seidler. London: Routledge, 1992. 1-26.

Sharpe, J. A. Early Modern England: A Social History 1550-1760. London: Edward Arnold, 1987.

Sherburn, George. Introduction. Caleb Williams. By William Godwin. New York: Holt, Rinehart & Winston, 1960. vii-xiv.

Siann, Gerda. Gender, Sex and Sexuality: Contemporary Psychological Perspectives. London: Taylor & Francis, 1994.

Silverman, Kaja. Male Subjectivity at the Margins. New York: Routledge, 1992.

Simms, Karl N. "Caleb Williams' Godwin: Things as they Are Written." Studies in Romanticism 26 (1987): 343-363.

Simpson, Mark. Male Impersonators: Men Performing Masculinity. London: Cassell, 1994.

Smith, Ken Edward. "William Godwin: Social Critique in Caleb Williams." Transactions of the Seventh International Congress on the Enlightenment. Vol. I. Ed. H. T. Mason. Oxford: The Voltaire Foundation, 1989. 337-341.

Spacks, Patricia Meyer. Desire and Truth. Chicago: U of Chicago P, 1990.

Spector, Robert Donald. The English Gothic: A Bibliographic Guide to Writers from Horace Walpole to Mary Shelley. Westport, CT: Greenwood, 1984.

Spencer, Jane. The Rise of the Woman Novelist: From Aphra Behn to Jane Austen. Oxford: Blackwell, 1986.

Spender, Dale. Mothers of the Novel: 100 Good Women Writers before Jane Austen. New York: Pandora, 1986.

Stevens, Cat. "Father and Son." Tea for the Tillerman. Beverly Hills, CA: A & M Records.

Stoller, Robert J. Sex and Gender: The Development of Masculinity and Feminity. Vol. 1. New York: Jason Aronson, 1968, 1974.

---. "The Term Perversion." Perversions and Near-Perversions in Clinical Practice: New Psychoanalytic Perspectives. Eds. Gerald I. Fogel and   Wayne A. Myers. New Haven: Yale UP, 1991. 36-56.

Stone, Lawrence. The Family, Sex and Marriage. New York: Harper, 1977.

---. The Past and Present Revisited. London: Routledge, 1981, 1987.

Storch, Rudolf F. "Metaphors of Private Guilt and Social Rebellion in Godwin's Caleb Williams." Journal of English Literary History 34 (1967): 188-207.

Straub, Kristina. Sexual Suspects: Eighteenth-Century Players and Sexual Ideology. Princeton: Princeton UP, 1992.

Summers, Monteque. The Gothic Quest. New York: Russell, 1964.

Tannahill, Reay. Sex in History. New York: Stein and Day, 1981.

Thomas, Calvin. Male Matters: Masculinity, Anxiety, and the Male Body on the Line. Urbana: U of Ill P, 1996.

Thompson, James. "Surveillance in William Godwin's Caleb Williams." Gothic Fictions: Prohibition/Transgression. Ed. Kenneth W. Graham. New York: AMS P, 1989. 173-198.

Thorslev, Peter. The Byronic Hero: Types and Prototypes. Minneapolis: U of Minnesota P, 1962.

Tolson, Andrew. The Limits of Masculinity: Male Identity and the Liberated Woman. New York: Harper & Row, 1977.

Troide, Lars E. Introduction. Horace Walpole's Miscellany 1786-1795. New Haven: Yale UP, 1978.

Trudgill, Eric. Madonnas and Magdalens: The Origins and Development of Victorian Sexual Attitudes. New York: Holmes & Meier, 1976.

Trumbach, Randolph. "London's Sodomites: Homosexual Behavior and Western Culture in Eighteenth Century. Journal of Social History 11 (1977): 1-33.

---. "The Birth of the Queen: Sodomy and the Emergence of Gender Equality in Modern Culture, 1660-1750." Hidden From History: Reclaiming the Gay and Lesbian Past. Eds. Martin Bauml Duberman et al. New York: NAL Books, 1989. 129-140.

Ty, Eleanor. Unsex'd Revolutionaries: Five Women Novelists of the 1790s. Toronto: U of Toronto P, 1993.

Varma, Devendra P. "Quest of the Numinous: The Gothic Flame." Literature of the Occult. Ed. Peter B. Messent. Englewood Cliffs, NJ: Prentice-Hall, 1981. 40-50.

---. The Gothic Flame. New York: Russell, 1966.

Varnado, S. L. Haunted Presence. Tuscaloosa: U of Alabama P, 1987.

Walpole, Horace. The Yale Edition of Horace Walpole's Correspondence. Vol. 10. Ed. W. S. Lewis. London: Humphrey Milford: Oxford UP, 1941.

---. The Castle of Otranto. Oxford: Oxford UP, 1982.

Warshow, Robert. "The Gangster as Tragic Hero." Reading Culture. Eds. Diana George and John Trimbur. 2nd ed. New York: HarperCollins, 1995. 374-377.

Watt, Ian. The Rise of the Novel: Studies in Defoe, Richardson and Fielding. Berkeley: U of Cal P, 1964.

Weber, Samuel. Return to Freud. Trans. Michael Levine. Cambridge: Cambridge UP, 1991.

Weeks, Jeffrey. Sex, Politics and Society: The Regulation of Sexuality Since 1800. London: Longman, 1981.

Williamson, Hugh Ross. The Day They Killed the King. London: Frederick Muller, 1957.

Wolstenholme, Susan. Gothic (Re)Visions: Writing Women as Readers. Albany: SUNY P, 1993.

Wollstonecraft, Mary. A Vindication of the Rights of Woman, A Mary Wollstonecraft Reader. Eds. Barbara H. Solomon and Paula S. Berggren. New York: Mentor, 1983.

Wordsworth, William. The Prose Works of William Wordsworth. Ed. W. J. B. Owen and Jane Worthington Smyser, Vol. 1, Oxford: Clarendon, 1974.

Yeasell, Ruth Bernard. Fictions of Modesty. Chicago: U of Chicago P, 1991.

Zizek, Slavoj. The Sublime Object of Ideology. London: Verso, 1989.

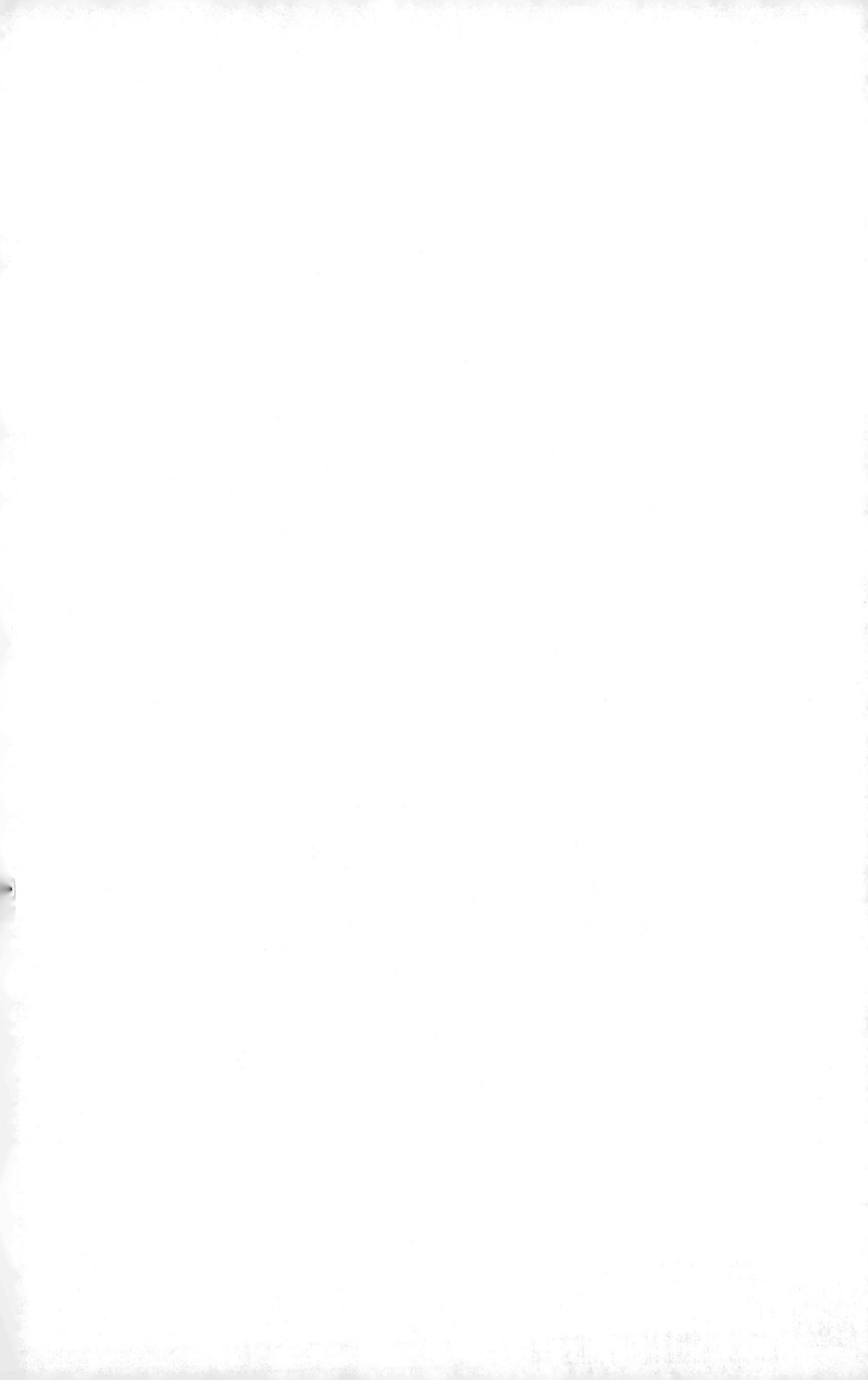

www.ingramcontent.com/pod-product-compliance
Lightning Source LLC
Chambersburg PA
CBHW021616270326
41931CB00008B/724